Emotional Well-Being Workbook

MIND-BODY WELLNESS SERIES

Facilitator Reproducible Sessions
for Motivated Behavior Modification

John J. Liptak, Ed.D.
Ester R.A. Leutenberg

Duluth, Minnesota

Whole Person
101 West 2nd St., Suite 203
Duluth, MN 55802

800-247-6789

books@wholeperson.com
www.wholeperson.com

Emotional Well-Being Workbook
Facilitator Reproducible Sessions
for Motivated Behavior Modification

Copyright ©2014 by John J. Liptak and Ester R.A. Leutenberg.
All rights reserved. Except for short excerpts for review purposes
and materials in the assessment, journaling activities, and
educational handouts sections, no part of this book may be
reproduced or transmitted in any form by any means, electronic
or mechanical without permission in writing from the publisher.
Self-assessments, exercises, and educational handouts are meant
to be photocopied.

All efforts have been made to ensure accuracy of the information
contained in this book as of the date published. The author(s)
and the publisher expressly disclaim responsibility for any
adverse effects arising from the use or application of the
information contained herein.

Printed in the United States of America

10 9 8 7 6 5 4 3 2 1

Editorial Director: Carlene Sippola
Art Director: Joy Morgan Dey

Library of Congress Control Number: 2013954249
ISBN: 978-1-57025-308-9

Our thanks to these professionals who make us look good!

Art Director – Joy Dey
Editor and Lifelong Teacher – Eileen Regen
Editorial Director – Carlene Sippola
Proofreader – Jay Leutenberg
Reviewer – Carol Butler

Introduction for the Facilitator

What is Emotional Well-Being?

Are your clients having difficulty understanding and expressing their emotions, feeling frustrated and angry but unable define why, living pessimistically and hopelessly, feeling inadequate for reasons they are unable to articulate, complaining about their inability to cope with the ups and downs of daily living, or acting scared at the thoughts of their lives changing? If so, they need to develop greater emotional wellness skills. Emotional wellness involves connecting your clients to their authentic emotions and helping them learn to deal with these emotions in healthy ways. *The Emotional Well-Being Workbook* is designed to help your clients connect with their emotions in a way that allows them to live an emotionally-balanced life.

Emotional well-being is related to how well your clients are able to express, understand, cope with, and manage their emotions. It reflects people who are aware of, and accepting of, their own emotions and the emotions of others. By reading this book and completing the assessments, activities, and exercises, your clients will benefit in the following ways:

- **Resilient** – They will be resistant from stress, guilt, anxiety, and depression.
- **Change** – They will be able to manage the uncertainty of change and transform their lives from the opportunities that change brings.
- **Self-Esteem** – They will be able to identify and operate from their strengths, with supreme confidence in their abilities.
- **Growth** – They will be able to harness the power of their emotions to grow personally and professionally.
- **Optimism** – They will begin to live their lives from the standpoint of positivity and possibility.

Living an emotionally well life does not mean that your clients will not experience stress, daily hassles, depression or life challenges. Like all people, they will continue to experience loss, grief, hardship, sadness and anxiety. The difference is that they will be armed with the knowledge, skills and abilities to deal effectively with whatever life throws at them. They will be positive people who have the ability to bounce back in the face of adversity. They will have the tools and techniques to cope with difficult life situations and maintain a positive outlook and positive sense of who they are as human beings.

Emotional Well-Being Workbook Sections

Observable actions and mannerisms that people display when reacting to particular stimuli are called behaviors. Behavior modification involves identifying ineffective behaviors, intentionally targeting them, setting goals for behavioral change, monitoring progress and determining effective rewards for improved behaviors.

The *Mind-Body Wellness Series* is composed of workbooks designed to help people learn how to discontinue old, destructive health habits and adopt new, healthy lifestyle choices. The model, referred to as Motivated Behavior Modification (MBM), looks at specific learned behaviors and the impact of environmental stimuli on those behaviors. It focuses on helping participants change undesirable and unhealthy lifestyle behaviors by objectively identifying unrealistic behaviors and replacing them with healthier, more effective behaviors.

Section 1 – Bounce Back

This chapter will help participants explore how effectively they bounce back from difficult situations and circumstances.

Section 2 – Identify and Express Emotions

This chapter will help participants explore how effectively they express their emotions to other people in their life.

Section 3 – Balance Work and Personal Life

This chapter will help participants determine how well they are living a balanced life.

Section 4 – Maintain a Hopeful Outlook

This chapter will help participants explore how hopeful they are about the future.

Section 5 – Feel Good About Yourself

This chapter will help participants explore how they feel about themselves.

Section 6 – Accept Change

This chapter will help participants explore how well they are able to be spontaneous when their lives change.

Section 7 – Enjoy Life, Laugh and Have Fun

This chapter helps participants explore how much fun and joy they are experiencing in life.

(Continued on the next page)

Changing Unhealthy Behaviors

Developing healthy emotions can be difficult, as implied in the adage "It's hard to teach an old dog new tricks!" Emotional well-being brings a sense of life satisfaction, joy and contentment. However, most people must work to develop healthy emotions and that is what this workbook does. This can be a challenging task for participants, but they can successfully change unhealthy emotions to healthier ones. This book uses a model known as MBM (Motivated Behavior Modification). For participants to be successful, you as the facilitator can enhance their motivation in several ways.

Components of Each Session

1. SELF-ASSESSMENT

Step 1 is the self-assessment of participants' current level of emotional well-being. Encourage participants to take one step at a time. By working on one set of behaviors at a time, the task of changing participant's behavior will not feel insurmountable. Because emotions can be difficult to enhance, it is important that they take small steps and work slowly to change how their emotions affect their lives. By trying to change more than one emotional characteristic at a time, people set themselves up for failure. Encourage participants to keep it simple! Each session is set up in a step format for the MBM of the emotions of each participant.

2. SUPPORT SYSTEM

Step 2 will guide participants to develop a support system of people who can help them achieve their goals of emotional well-being. Encourage participants to develop a support system to help them be more emotionally resilient. It is important that you encourage participants to define who in their lives can help and support them while they develop the emotions that accompany a bounce-back attitude. Encourage participants to let people know that they are trying to change the emotions they experience and express that they don't have to suffer in silence. Explain that each participant's support system will vary for each type of behavior.

3. JOURNALING

Step 3 includes journaling questions to help participants reflect about their emotional reactions in the past. Encourage participants to write everything down in a journal. Remind them that words are shallow and just saying they are going to make changes will not suffice. Journaling can be therapeutic as well as a way to begin identifying goals for greater emotional well-being.

4. GOAL-SETTING

Step 4 will remind participants not to give up and to be persistent in their efforts to make emotional growth. Explain that this takes time and that they should not expect immediate results. The purpose of setting goals is to help each participant take smaller steps leading to the selected overall goal. Encourage them to review and revise their plans to build resilient, positive emotions and attitudes. By developing MBM goals to work toward and achieve, participants will remain motivated while they slowly learn how to identify and express their emotions.

5. MONITORING MY BEHAVIOR

Step 5 will help participants to see the progress they are making in developing emotional competency. This will assist participants to be accountable, persistent, and motivated to make emotional changes. You should act as coach and encourage participants to develop and utilize their newfound emotional attitudes.

6. REWARD YOURSELF

Step 6 will ensure that participants reward themselves as they achieve their emotional goals. Remind participants to reward themselves when they do improve. HEALTHY rewards provide them with positive feedback and further motivate them to continue creating their own emotional well-being.

7. TIPS

Step 7 Participants will grow from reading and implementing the various tips which are included as suggestions for processing each session.

(Continued on the next page)

Motivational Barriers to Behavioral Change

Emotions can hinder behavioral change and many of these barriers show up in peoples' emotions. The impact of emotions on a person's motivation and subsequent behavioral changes can be monumental. Therefore, as the facilitator, it will help to be aware of any emotional barriers that may be keeping participants from being successful as they work to live happier, emotionally-well lives.

Following are some of the most prominent reasons that bar people from changing their negative, pessimistic emotions into positive, hopeful, and optimistic ones.

- Some people prefer instant gratification and fail to look at the long-term benefits and consequences of their behavior. People who work too much are often too worried about climbing the corporate ladder to see the effects their workaholic lifestyle is having on their emotions and the emotions of members of their family. They, and the members of their family, probably feel frustrated, stressed, and upset.

- Some people continue to experience negative emotions, often thinking that they will deal with the consequences at a later date. People unable to experience work-life balance find themselves being so negative that they alienate everyone around them.

- Some people feel they are too busy to worry about the consequences of unhealthy emotions. Because they are so wrapped up in work, they don't see or care that they are being negative and pessimistic.

- Some people simply are indifferent to unhealthy behaviors. They will express such negative ideas as *"This will never work out"* or *"You won't be able to do it!"*

- Some people have a sense of invincibility and believe that negative emotions will not affect them. A workaholic will say such things as "I am not grouchy" although they are constantly yelling at significant others in their lives.

Enhanced emotional well-being has been shown to contribute to one's ability to cope with stressors and change in life, self-esteem, and longevity. In working with emotions to enhance emotional well-being, you need to remember that emotions can influence thoughts and behaviors.

It is important to understand emotions and the ways in which thoughts and perceptions can alter the emotions people experience. Emotions have the quality of alerting people that something is wrong in their lives and something needs to be changed.

This workbook is designed to help your participants explore their negative emotions, identify why they are feeling these emotions, and explore ways to change negative emotions into positive ones.

(Continued on the next page)

Using this Workbook to Modify Behavior

Behavior Modification programs provide a process to PERMANENTLY change destructive and negative emotions and replace them with positive ones that will lead to greater health and well-being. The behavior modification program included in this series of workbooks contains several critical components:

Motivated Behavior Modification (MBM) Components

STEP 1: Self-Assessment – The first step in modifying behavior involves determining the frequency, circumstances, and outcomes of the emotions to be altered or enhanced. MBM relies on objective self-assessment to determine each participant's unhealthy emotions and to establish a baseline for their strengths and limitations. Once a baseline is established, the data collected can be used to track a participant's progress in changing unhealthy emotions to more healthy ones. The self-assessments contained in this workbook are referred to as "formative assessments" and can be used to assess participant's current level of functioning and also to measure emotional change over time.

In this stage, people acknowledge that they have a problem and begin to seriously think about making healthier lifestyle changes. They want to explore in depth the level of their difficulties in changing negative emotions. Self-assessments are very powerful tools for helping participants learn more about themselves to gain valuable insights into their constructive and destructive emotions. Self-assessments are used by participants to better understand themselves and gain valuable insights into their thinking, feelings and behaviors. Self-assessments allow facilitators to gather information about participants to get a complete picture of each person.

Facts about self-assessments:

- Self-assessments provide you with a small sample of behavior and should not be used to stereotype participants. Self-assessments are designed to allow participants to explore their behavioral strengths and weaknesses.

- Factors such as cultural background, handicaps, and age should be taken into consideration when exploring self-assessment results.

- Self-assessments are designed to be self-administered, scored and interpreted by the participants. However, facilitators should be available to assist participants in understanding their scores in an objective and helpful way.

- Self-assessments are designed to gather self-reported data, thus the results are dependent on each participant's motivation and cooperation.

- Self-assessment results should be explored in light of other behavioral data facilitators have available, not in isolation.

- Self-assessments can be used with individual participants or with groups.

- Self-assessments can be used to form specific decisions about the type of instruction that would be most beneficial. Thus, if your group scores lowest on a particular self-assessment for a chapter, that might be an effective place to concentrate instruction.

- Participants can use the results of their self-assessments to adjust and improve their behavior.

(Continued on the next page)

Using this Workbook to Modify Behavior
Motivated Behavior Modification (MBM) Components *(Continued)*

STEP 2: Support System – The next step in behavior modification involves participants recognizing who is in their support system and identifying which people are supportive of which topics. This requires participants to think about who can support them through each particular behavior modification, what their supporters can do, and how they will help. Support people may vary for each behavior. The person who is being supportive about low self-esteem can be different from the one being supportive about balancing work and personal life.

STEP 3: Journaling – The next step in behavior modification is journaling answers to specific questions. Journaling has been shown to be very effective in helping people to think critically about themselves and issues they are coping with. It is wise to remind participants not to concern themselves with grammar or spelling. Just free-writing thoughts and ideas is the purpose of the journal.

STEP 4: Goal Setting – The next step in behavior modification is to set goals to modify behavior. Goals initiate an action plan and are necessary to motivate behavioral change. Participants will set goals that will replace their old, negative habits with new, healthier habits. It is important to help participants determine which specific behaviors they want to change. This will help to give order and context to the change process. Goals provide participants with direction, priorities and a well-conceived action plan for MBM. Goals should meet these criteria:

- **Specific and Behavioral:** Goals must be stated in concrete, behavioral terms. For example, "I would like to be able to maintain emotional balance when I am experiencing change in my life" would be a concrete, behavioral goal.
- **Measurable:** Goals must be measurable so that people can track their progress. For example, "during an upcoming change in my life, I will meditate daily and look for opportunities in the change".
- **Attainable:** Goals must be within reach or participants will not be motivated to work toward them. They must feel that they have a realistic opportunity to achieve their goals. For example, "By setting aside 15 minutes each night to meditate and reflect on the change in my life, I will be able to maintain emotional balance."
- **Relevant:** Goals must be important to the participant. For example, knowing that a person who is feeling emotional balance will be able to maintain harmony at home.
- **Time-Specific:** Goals must have specific times for completion if they are going to have power. However, the time frames need to be reasonable and realistic so that participants will feel committed. For example, by setting a goal of "within the next week, I will begin setting 15 minutes aside to meditate and reflect," the person will set a specific time within which to begin developing emotional balance.

The goal setting process helps participants to be personally accountable in changing their unhealthy behaviors.

STEP 5: Monitoring – The next step is to monitor behaviors until desired outcomes are reached. Sections will be included for participants to keep a regular record of their activities and progress. Motivation is the intrinsic drive that pushes participants into action and makes permanent behavioral changes. Motivation is enhanced when participants are working toward specific goals and monitoring their progress as they continue to make motivated behavioral modifications. By monitoring their progress as they move toward goals, participants reinforce MBM.

STEP 6: Rewards – This step defines rewards for accomplishing behavioral goals. Healthy rewards will vary from person to person. Participants will benefit by rewarding themselves for any positive steps taken to change unhealthy behaviors.

STEP 7: Tips – This final step provides insights into ways people can deal with unwanted behaviors.

Introduction for the Participant

Most major emotional problems today are due to an inability to understand and express feelings, feel comfortable with those feelings, and achieve emotional stability. When you are able to understand and take responsibility for the way you express your own emotions, you are then able to understand and accept the emotions of others. This ability is critical in developing and maintaining effective, healthy relationships.

Emotional wellness is very important to your overall well-being. People who are emotionally well tend to be able to understand and express their emotions and the effect of their emotions on others. They are more likely to be free of worry and anxiety, maintain an optimistic life outlook regardless of the events occurring in their lives, are able to overcome frustrations that occur, work to live happy lives, and take time out to laugh and engage in their favorite activities.

There are many benefits from maintaining emotional wellness:

- Ability to express emotions effectively.
- Adjust to change.
- Cope with uncomfortable emotions in healthier ways.
- Enjoy life despite its disappointments and frustrations.
- Appreciate healthy relationships.
- Focus in the present and not fear the future.
- Bounce back when experiencing different situations.
- Feelings of joy.
- Feel good about yourself.

As you can see, there are many reasons to develop emotional wellness skills and habits.

The biggest challenge is finding ways to identify and express your own emotions and recognize emotions of others so that you can develop healthy relationships.

The purpose of the *Emotional Well-Being Workbook* is to help you understand the relationship between emotions and your overall well-being and keep you motivated while you modify your emotional behavior. In this workbook, you will engage in various types of self-assessments, have an opportunity to set effective emotional goals, and look forward to living a healthier life.

(Continued on the next page)

EMOTIONAL WELL-BEING

Introduction for the Participant *(Continued)*

Some Things to Remember

Developing healthy lifestyle choices can be difficult, as is implied in the adage "It's difficult to teach an old dog new tricks!" Developing positive emotions can be a challenging task, but successfully changing your negative emotions to positive emotions can be accomplished.

You can do this!

- Take one step at a time. By working on one behavior at a time, the task of changing your behavior will not feel insurmountable. Because emotions are so difficult to change, it is important to start with small emotions and work slowly to change one at a time. By trying to change more than one behavior at a time, people set themselves up for failure. Keep it simple!

- Create a support system to help you change your emotions. Who can you ask for help and support in changing your unhealthy emotions? Choose people with whom you feel comfortable, and people who would be helpful in a specific area of your life who know that you are trying to make changes. You don't have to suffer in silence to successfully change an unhealthy emotion to a healthy one. Let people know about your desire to change and allow others to support you.

- Write everything down on paper. Saying you are going to make changes will not suffice. Self-assessments, working on defined behaviors and writing concrete goals will help you to be successful.

- Be persistent in your effort and do not to give up on yourself. Remember that it takes time to change emotional patterns. Do not expect immediate results. The purpose of setting goals is to help you take smaller steps leading to your overall goal. Plan for a healthier lifestyle. By developing motivated behavior modification (MBM) goals to work toward and achieve, you will remain motivated while you slowly turn unhealthy habits into healthy ones.

- Be accountable. If during your efforts to make positive changes you slip and go back to old emotional habits, don't let this stop you. Attempt to learn from your setbacks and use your newfound knowledge to make successful choices. Monitor our progress.

- Reward yourself for a job well done. HEALTHY rewards provide you with positive feedback and motivate you to continue in your efforts to develop greater emotional well-being. You will find ways to reward yourself for a job well done!

- Use the tips, as applicable to you, provided on the last page of each of the sessions.

You are now prepared to begin making motivated behavior modifications (MBMs)! Working through the steps in each session of this workbook will allow you to more easily change unhealthy emotions into more healthy ones. This process really works. It is an exciting way to change your emotions and begin to enjoy and appreciate a happier, healthier life.

Table of Contents

Section I – Bounce Back
- Step 1: Self-Assessment Introduction and Directions 17
  - Self-Assessment 18
  - Self-Assessment Scoring Directions 19
  - Self-Assessment Profile Interpretation 19
  - Self-Assessment Descriptions 20
- Step 2: Recognize and Develop a Support System 20
- Step 3: Keep a Journal – Difficult Situations 21
- Step 4: Set Goals 22
- Step 5: Monitor My Behavior – Believe Success is Possible 23–24
  - Monitor My Behavior – Remain Open Minded 25–26
  - Monitor My Behavior – Have a Positive Sense of Self 27–28
- Step 6: Reward Myself 29
- Step 7: Tips for Motivated Behavior Modifications 30

Section II – Identify and Express Emotions
- Step 1: Self-Assessment Introduction and Directions 33
  - Self-Assessment 34
  - Self-Assessment Scoring Directions 35
  - Self-Assessment Profile Interpretation 35
  - Self-Assessment Descriptions 36
- Step 2: Recognize and Develop a Support System 36
- Step 3: Keep a Journal 37
  - Keep a Journal of My Emotions 38
- Step 4: Set Goals 39
- Step 5: Monitor My Behavior – Awareness 40
  - Monitor My Behavior – Body Language 41
  - Monitor My Behavior – Direct 42
- Step 6: Reward Myself 43
- Step 7: Tips for Motivated Behavior Modifications 44

Section III – Balance Work and Personal Life
- Step 1: Self-Assessment Introduction and Directions 47
  - Self-Assessment 48
  - Self-Assessment Scoring Directions 49
  - Self-Assessment Profile Interpretation 49
  - Self-Assessment Descriptions 49
- Step 2: Recognize and Develop a Support System 50
- Step 3: Keep a Journal 51
- Step 4: Set Goals 52
- Step 5: Monitor My Behavior – Work Life 53–54
  - Monitor My Behavior – Personal Life 55–56
- Step 6: Reward Myself 57
- Step 7: Tips for Motivated Behavior Modifications 58

(Continued)

Table of Contents

Section IV – Maintain a Hopeful Outlook
- Step 1: Self-Assessment Introduction and Directions ... 61
  - Self-Assessment ... 62–63
  - Self-Assessment Scoring Directions ... 64
  - Self-Assessment Profile Interpretation ... 65
- Step 2: Recognize and Develop a Support System ... 65
- Step 3: Keep a Journal ... 66
- Step 4: Set Goals ... 67
- Step 5: Monitor My Behavior – Hope ... 68
  - Monitor My Behavior – Life Outlook ... 69
  - Monitor My Behavior – Attitude ... 70
  - Overcoming Obstacles ... 71
- Step 6: Reward Myself ... 72
- Step 7: Tips for Motivated Behavior Modifications ... 73

Section V – Feel Good About Yourself
- Step 1: Self-Assessment Introduction and Directions ... 77
  - Self-Assessment ... 78–79
  - Self-Assessment Scoring Directions ... 80
  - Self-Assessment Profile Interpretation ... 80
  - Self-Assessment Descriptions ... 81
- Step 2: Recognize and Develop a Support System ... 81
- Step 3: Keep a Journal ... 82
- Step 4: Set Goals ... 83
- Step 5: Monitor My Behavior – Pride ... 84
- Step 5: Monitor My Behavior – Image ... 85
- Step 5: Monitor My Behavior – Outlook ... 86
- Step 5: Monitor My Behavior – Self-Approval ... 87
- Step 5: Monitor My Behavior – Summary ... 88
- Step 6: Reward Myself ... 89
- Step 7: Tips for Motivated Behavior Modifications ... 90

Section VI – Accept Change
- Step 1: Self-Assessment Introduction and Directions ... 93
  - Self-Assessment ... 94
  - Self-Assessment Scoring Directions ... 95
  - Self-Assessment Profile Interpretation ... 95
- Step 2: Recognize and Develop a Support System ... 96
- Step 3: Keep a Journal ... 97
- Step 4: Set Goals ... 98
- Step 5: Monitor My Behavior – Realistic ... 99–100
  - Monitor My Behavior – Wellness ... 101–102
  - Monitor My Behavior – Control ... 103–104
- Step 6: Reward Myself ... 105
- Step 7: Tips for Motivated Behavior Modifications ... 106

(Continued)

Table of Contents

Section VII – Enjoy Life, Laugh and Have Fun
    Step 1: Self-Assessment Introduction and Directions.................................109
        Self-Assessment...110–112
        Self-Assessment Scoring Directions..113
        Self-Assessment Profile Interpretation......................................113
        Self-Assessment Descriptions...114
    Step 2: Recognize and Develop a Support System...................................114
    Step 3: Keep a Journal..115
    Step 4: Set Goals...116
    Step 5: Monitor My Behavior – Enjoy Life....................................117–118
        Monitor My Behavior – Laugh...119–120
        Monitor My Behavior – Have Fun..121–122
    Step 6: Reward Myself...123
    Step 7: Tips for Motivated Behavior Modifications.................................124

SECTION I

BOUNCE BACK

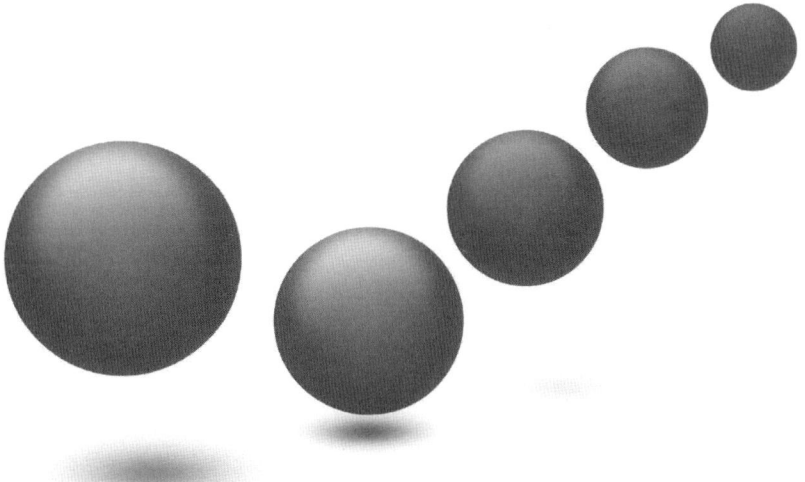

"No matter how far life pushes you down, no matter how much you hurt, you can always bounce back."

— **Sheryl Swoops**

Name _____

Date _____

EMOTIONAL WELL-BEING

EMOTIONAL WELL-BEING

BOUNCE BACK

Step 1: Self-Assessment Introduction and Directions

Resiliency is the ability to bounce back when the going gets tough. A resilient person is able to handle hardship and turn setbacks into comebacks, regain stability quickly in difficult situations and stay emotionally healthy during periods of uncertainty and stress. They are able to rebound from adversity even healthier than they were.

The purpose of the Bounce Back Self-Assessment is to help you explore how resilient you are in times of difficulty and stress. Read each statement carefully and circle the number of the response that describes you best.

	USUALLY TRUE	RARELY TRUE	NOT TRUE
1. I see challenges as interesting opportunities	(3)	2	1

In the above example, the circled 3 indicates that the responder usually sees challenges as interesting opportunities.

This is not a test and there are no right or wrong answers. Do not spend too much time thinking about your answers. Your initial response will be the most true for you. Be sure to respond to every statement.

Turn the page and complete the Self-Assessment

EMOTIONAL WELL-BEING

BOUNCE BACK

Step 1: Self-Assessment

	USUALLY TRUE	RARELY TRUE	NOT TRUE
1. I see challenges as interesting opportunities	3	2	1
2. I expect things to work out	3	2	1
3. I can't find solutions to problems in times of trouble	1	2	3
4. I expect the best for myself and others	3	2	1
5. I am able to view stressful situations as personal challenges	3	2	1
6. I wonder why terrible things keep happening to me	1	2	3
7. I know that bad things will happen to me	1	2	3
8. I am able to ignore hurtful criticism	3	2	1
9. I know I can make good things happen in my life	3	2	1
10. I believe that I will be successful	3	2	1

I. TOTAL = _____

11. I am open-minded to new ideas	3	2	1
12. I am not very flexible or adaptable	1	2	3
13. I have a difficult time with change	3	2	1
14. I am not spontaneous	1	2	3
15. I use humor to help me through tough times	3	2	1
16. Not knowing what's in store for me in the future does not bother me	3	2	1
17. I have trouble taking positive, calculated risks	1	2	3
18. I am able to make light of myself even in difficult situations	3	2	1
19. I have a hard time motivating myself	1	2	3
20. I am able to bounce back when situations get tough	3	2	1

II. TOTAL = _____

21. I recognize my special talents	3	2	1
22. I have focus in my life	3	2	1
23. I want to make a positive contribution to society	3	2	1
24. I worry about what my peers say about me	1	2	3
25. I take responsibility for my actions	3	2	1
26. I like to discover new things about myself, positive or negative	3	2	1
27. I do not give up on anything until it is completed	3	2	1
28. I feel like I am a victim	1	2	3
29. I am able to learn from my mistakes	3	2	1
30. I worry about looking foolish in front of anyone	1	2	3

III. TOTAL = _____

Go to the Scoring Directions on the next page

EMOTIONAL WELL-BEING

BOUNCE BACK

Step 1: Self Assessment Scoring Directions

The self-assessment you just completed is designed to help you explore whether you to bounce back from difficult situations or when the going gets tough. For each of the items on the previous page, total the scores you circled. Add your circled numbers and put that total on the line marked TOTAL at the end of the section and then transfer that number below.

_____ I. Believe Success is Possible

_____ II. Remain Open-Minded

_____ III. Have a Positive Sense-of-Self

Profile Interpretation

Find the range for your scores and use the information below to assist you in the interpretation of your scores.

Total Scales Scores	Result	Indications
Scores from 24 to 30	High	You are able to easily bounce-back when times get tough. You believe that great things are going to happen, you are very open-minded and have an excellent sense of yourself.
Scores from 17 to 23	Moderate	You are somewhat able to bounce-back when times get tough. You believe that good things are going to happen, you are open-minded and have a positive sense of yourself.
Scores from 10 to 16	Low	You have a difficult time bouncing-back when times get tough. You do not believe that good things are going to happen, you are not very open-minded, and have a do not have a positive sense of yourself.

Go to the Scale Descriptions on the next page

EMOTIONAL WELL-BEING

BOUNCE BACK

Step 1: Self-Assessment Descriptions

Believe Success is Possible – This self-assessment is designed to measure your level of resilient thinking. People scoring high on this self-assessment usually have a positive belief system. They look for what's right rather than what's wrong. They believe that they are going to be successful.

Remain Open-Minded – This self-assessment is designed to measure how open-minded you are. People scoring high on this self-assessment are usually flexible and can adapt to different situations easily. They are receptive to new ideas and are not bothered by uncertainty.

Have a Positive Sense of Self – This self-assessment is designed to measure how well you know yourself. People scoring high on this self-assessment usually understand and utilize their talents and special skills. They are not worried about what others think of them and they take responsibility for making sure that good things happen in their lives.

Step 2: Recognize and Develop a Support System

To bounce back in difficult times, a support system can be critical in your success. Not every supportive person in your life will be helpful, but many will be supportive. Complete the following table with people who might be able to support you with your ability to bounce back from difficulties.

Supporter	How This Person Can Support Me	How I Can Contact This Person
My friend Sally	She is good at reminding me of my special qualities	Email: Sally@.com, Phone and Text: 000-0000

Keep this list handy. Call, email or text when you need support.

BOUNCE BACK

Step 3: Keep a Journal – Difficult Situations

The following journaling questions are designed to help you develop and maintain a resilient outlook and prepare you to be able to bounce back from difficult situations. Remember, your thinking can affect how motivated you are to make healthy changes in your behavior.

What difficult situations do you face in your life?

_____

_____

_____

How are you handling them?

_____

_____

_____

What difficult situations have you faced in the past?

_____

_____

_____

How have you handled them?

_____

_____

_____

What keeps you from bouncing back from difficult situations?

_____

_____

_____

EMOTIONAL WELL-BEING

BOUNCE BACK

Step 4: Set Goals

A well-conceived action plan will help you to develop the resiliency skills to help you cope with stress and adversity. For your action plan identify both the behavior you want to change and the goals required for you to reach the ultimate goals that will help you to bounce back easily and quickly.

The behavior I want to change _____

Goals need to be SMART:
Specific, **M**easureable, **A**ttainable, **R**ealistic and **T**ime-Specific

Goals	How I Will Measure This Goal	How Is This Goal Attainable and Realistic?	Time Deadline	How This Will Help Me
Have less arguments with members of my blended family	Less amount of verbal confrontations	I can be more flexible and open-minded with ALL family members.	6 months	I will have less stress and more family harmony.

If you are having trouble identifying goals, consult TIPS, page 30.

EMOTIONAL WELL-BEING

BOUNCE BACK

Step 5: Monitor My Behavior – Believe Success is Possible

Monitoring your progress toward your resiliency goals will help ensure that the ability to bounce back becomes a part of your personality. Keeping track of your behaviors through logs will help you determine what you have accomplished at given times. Periodic re-evaluations support your success. Once you reach your goal(s), set new ones to improve or maintain what you have already achieved. Use a separate page for each bounce back behavior you want to improve.

EXAMPLE:

My healthy behavior change Have a more positive outlook in life

My goal See opportunities for improving my life after being downsized

Date	My Accomplishment	How It Felt
1/1/2014	I made an effort to see new job possibilities.	I feel a new energy and excitement.

Believe Success is Possible

My healthy behavior change _____

My goal _____

Date	My Accomplishment	How It Felt

(Continued on the next page)

EMOTIONAL WELL-BEING

BOUNCE BACK

Step 5: Monitor My Behavior
Believe Success is Possible *(Continued)*

Write about a setback you have encountered lately?

_____
_____
_____
_____
_____

What keeps you from believing you can be successful after experiencing this setback?

_____
_____
_____
_____
_____

How can you begin to see the opportunities in this situations?

_____
_____
_____
_____
_____

How can you begin to make positive things happen?

_____
_____
_____
_____
_____

(Continued on the next page)

EMOTIONAL WELL-BEING

BOUNCE BACK

Step 5: Monitor My Behavior – Remain Open Minded

Monitoring your progress toward your goals will help to develop and maintain a more open-minded outlook on life. Keeping track of your behaviors through logs will help you determine what you have accomplished at given times. Periodic re-evaluations support your success. Once you reach your goal(s), set new ones to improve your ability to bounce back. Use a separate page for each change.

EXAMPLE:

My healthy behavior change Lighten up a bit

My goal Not get frustrated by life's little frustrations

Date	My Accomplishment	How It Felt
1/1/2014	I didn't become angry when the garage door wouldn't open.	It felt good to be not so quick to anger.

Remain Open Minded

My healthy behavior change _____

My goal _____

Date	My Accomplishment	How It Felt

(Continued on the next page)

EMOTIONAL WELL-BEING

BOUNCE BACK

Step 5: Monitor My Behavior – Remain Open Minded *(Continued)*

How can you live your life more spontaneously?

_____
_____
_____
_____
_____

In what ways are you flexible? Rigid?

_____
_____
_____
_____
_____

What types of healthy, calculated risks do you want to begin taking?

_____
_____
_____
_____
_____

How can you incorporate more laughter into your life?

_____
_____
_____
_____
_____

(Continued on the next page)

EMOTIONAL WELL-BEING

BOUNCE BACK

Step 5: Monitor My Behavior – Have a Positive Sense of Self

A positive sense of self is critical in bouncing back! Monitoring your progress toward your goals will help to reinforce your resiliency. Keeping track of your behaviors through logs will help you determine what you have accomplished at given times. Periodic re-evaluations support your success. As you achieve your resiliency goals, set new ones to improve or maintain what you have already achieved. Use a separate page for each way you want to develop greater resiliency.

EXAMPLE:

My healthy behavior change To begin using my talents more

My goal To start writing again, even if I don't show it to anyone

Date	My Accomplishment	How It Felt
1/1/2014	I wrote ten pages.	Satisfying.

Have a Positive Sense of Self

My healthy behavior change _____

My goal _____

Date	My Accomplishment	How It Felt

(Continued on the next page)

EMOTIONAL WELL-BEING

BOUNCE BACK

Step 5: Monitor My Behavior
Have a Positive Sense of Self (Continued)

What talents do you possess that you use now? _____
_____
_____

What talents do you possess that you don't use? _____
_____
_____

Why don't you use these talents? _____
_____
_____

When do you find yourself feeling like a victim? _____
_____
_____

How can you overcome those feelings? _____
_____
_____

About what would you like to learn? _____
_____
_____

What are you doing when you are most worried about what other people say? _____
_____
_____

Do you really need to care? Why or Why not? _____
_____
_____

EMOTIONAL WELL-BEING

BOUNCE BACK

Step 6: Reward Myself

You now are beginning to bounce back from adversity! Congratulations! You need to give yourself a pat on the back or some other reward. People who reward themselves are more likely to remain resilient than people who don't! Your reward needs to be something that will give you the incentive to bounce back more quickly and easily. It needs to be healthy, within your budget and something you'll be excited about. If you are buying yourself something, be sure your reward is something you wouldn't ordinarily buy or do. Brainstorm some possible rewards.

- Rewards that would be meaningful to me _____
- Small rewards I could give myself _____
- Large rewards I could give myself _____
- Things that would not cost money and would be fun _____
- Rewards that I can afford and that would be fun _____
- Rewards that I enjoy alone _____
- Rewards I enjoy with people who support me _____

You deserve a pat on the back for the hard work you are completing in this session. Rewards help you to pay attention to your triumphs, not your setbacks. Rewards will create good feelings and propel you to want to work harder to reach your goals. Whenever you have completed or achieved one of your goals, treat yourself to one of the items on your list. You can also reward yourself by giving yourself positive affirmations when you have achieved a goal. Below are some samples. Cut them out and post in visible spots at home and work! If these don't work for your goal, write your own on sticky notes!

I am creative and resourceful.	Good things do happen to me!	I have control over my own thoughts.
I know that I will be okay!	*I'm sure things will work out for me!*	I am emotionally resilient!
I choose to have a positive attitude.	**I bounce back when things get tough!**	*I am open-minded!*

Pablo Valle said, "Write this down: My life is full of unlimited possibilities."
What are the possibilities in your life? List them.

_____
_____

EMOTIONAL WELL-BEING

BOUNCE BACK

Step 7: Tips For Motivated Behavior Modifications

Believe Success is Possible

- Use positive thinking such as *"I am responsible for my own success"* and *"I can turn this setback into an opportunity"* in the face of setbacks.

- Set and work toward goals and you will be successful.

- Build on your positive, uplifting successes from the past. Think about how you can replicate the process.

- Identify exciting challenges that may be hiding in the difficulties you face.

Open-Mindedness

- Stay hungry for opportunities to stretch yourself and learn new things. What would you like to learn more about?

- Lighten up by incorporating humor into your life. Try going to a silly movie, reading a funny book or magazine, or recall funny jokes you have heard or incidents from the past.

- Take positive, calculated risks that stretch beyond your comfort level.

- Find ways to enjoy the mystery of not knowing almost as much as you enjoy definitiveness and certainty.

Positive Sense of Self

- Know and understand your limitations and work to overcome them. You can also try to use your limitation in a novel and creative way.

- Maintain focus and a sense of purpose in your life.

- Identify and explore your philosophical framework through which difficult personal experiences can be interpreted with meaning and hope.

- Learn from your mistakes. Think about several things you did in the past that you feel were mistakes. Describe what you learned from these experiences. How will this understanding help you in the future?

SECTION II

IDENTIFY AND EXPRESS EMOTIONS

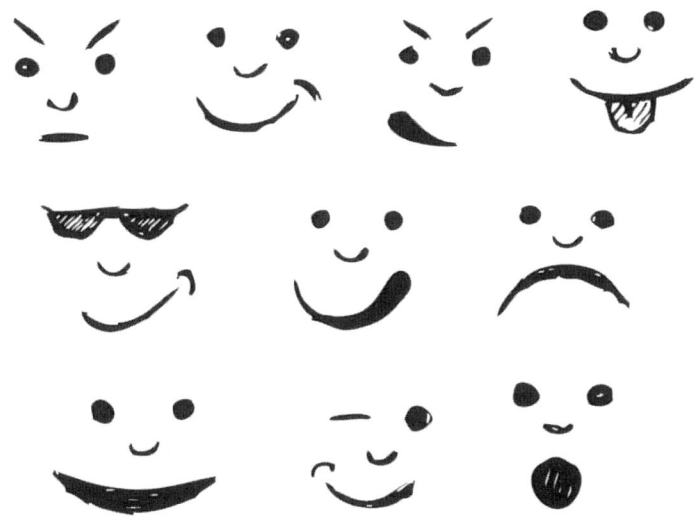

"They may forget what you said, but they will never forget how you made them feel."

~ Carl W. Buechner

Name _____

Date _____

EMOTIONAL WELL-BEING

EMOTIONAL WELL-BEING

IDENTIFY and EXPRESS EMOTIONS

Step 1: Self-Assessment Introduction and Directions

Emotions often need to be dealt with and your ability to express those emotions to other people effectively is one of the most important aspects of emotional well-being. To maintain emotional wellness, you need to be able to identify your emotions, understand your own body language and express emotions to other people. The *Identify and Express Emotions Scale* was designed to help you examine how well you are at identifying and expressing your emotions.

This self-assessment contains 18 statements related to the exchange-of-information. Read each of the statements and decide whether or not the statement describes you. If the statement is true, circle the number next to that item under the TRUE column. If the statement is false, circle the number next to that item under the FALSE column.

In the following example, the circled number under FALSE indicates the statement is not true of the person completing the inventory.

	TRUE	FALSE
When I am expressing my emotions to another person ...		
I have a difficult time understanding what I'm feeling.	1	(2)

This is not a test and there are no right or wrong answers. Do not spend too much time thinking about your answers. Your initial response will likely be the most true for you. Be sure to respond to every statement.

Turn the page and complete the Self-Assessment

EMOTIONAL WELL-BEING

IDENTIFY and EXPRESS EMOTIONS

Step 1: Self-Assessment

	TRUE	FALSE
When I am expressing my emotions to another person ...		
I have a difficult time understanding what I'm feeling	1	2
I understand my feelings and express them so they are not misunderstood	2	1
I often am not sure what I'm feeling so I can't explain it to anyone else	1	2
I tend to stuff my emotions rather than disclose them	1	2
I don't understand my feelings, so I ignore them	1	2
I am aware of, and own, my feelings	2	1

A – TOTAL = _____

I look the other person in the eye	2	1
I am not aware of the messages my body sends	1	2
I keep my body posture open to the other person	2	1
I lean a little toward the person who is speaking	2	1
I rarely nod my head to show understanding	1	2
I tend to look around when another person is talking	1	2

B – TOTAL = _____

I find it difficult always get to the point quickly	1	2
I am aware of how my tone and volume affects my messages	2	1
I express my feelings by starting with *"I feel __"*	2	1
I rarely check to make sure the other person understands	1	2
I am assertive, but not passive or aggressive	2	1
I am calm, open and direct when talking to another person	2	1

D – TOTAL = _____

Go to the Scoring Directions on the next page

EMOTIONAL WELL-BEING

IDENTIFY and EXPRESS EMOTIONS

Step 1: Self Assessment Scoring Directions

Many people are not always willing or able to express their emotions, however it is a skill that can be learned. This self-assessment is designed to measure how effectively you communicate your emotions to other people. At the bottom of each of the categories on the previous page, add the numbers that you circled. Then transfer your totals below.

    A – Awareness   Total = _____

    B – Body Language Total = _____

    D – Direct   Total = _____

Now add your three scores together to get your Grand Total and put that number below:

    GRAND TOTAL   = _____

Profile Interpretation

Individual Scales Scores	Grand Total	Result	Indications
11 to 12	31 to 36	High	**If you scored between 11 and 12 on any scale**, you are effective in expressing your emotions to other people. Keep up the good work!
8 to 10	24 to 30	Moderate	**If you scored between 8 and 10**, you are fairly effective in expressing your emotions to other people. Continue working to improve your effectiveness.
6 to 7	18 to 23	Low	**If your score was between 6 and 7**, you are not very effective in expressing your emotions to other people. You should work to improve your skills.

Go to the Scale Descriptions on the next page

EMOTIONAL WELL-BEING

IDENTIFY and EXPRESS EMOTIONS

Step 1: Self-Assessment Descriptions

Awareness – People scoring high on this scale are skilled at clearly understanding what they are feeling. Because they fully understand their emotions, they are effective in conveying their emotions. They rarely ignore or repress their emotions because they know they are expressing what they truly feel.

Body Language – Your body language can say as much as your words say. People scoring high on this scale understand that it is important to be aware of how body language is sending messages consistent with the tone of the discussion. They also pay attention to the body language of other people that allows them to better understand what other people are feeling.

Direct – People scoring high on this scale are skilled at getting their messages across to other people in an honest, open and direct way. They do not "beat around the bush" and are assertive in expressing their messages. They keep their messages simple and clear.

Step 2: Recognize and Develop a Support System

In order to effectively address and express your various emotions, you need people who will support you and be available to you when you need them. Not every person in your life will be helpful for each of your challenges. Complete the following table with people who might be able to support you in expressing your emotions effectively.

Supporter	How This Person Can Support Me	How I Can Contact This Person
My friend Nellie	By reminding me to open up and express myself when I'm feeling emotional	Phone only: 123-4567

Keep this list handy. Call, email or text when you need support.

EMOTIONAL WELL-BEING

IDENTIFY and EXPRESS EMOTIONS

Step 3: Keep a Journal

Reflecting on and journaling about how you express emotions in your life can be therapeutic. Following are some journaling exercises that can help you think thoroughly about the behaviors related to expressing emotions that you need to change. Remember, your thinking can affect how well you are able to express your emotions to other people in your life.

When is it difficult to express your emotions to other people?

___

Why is it difficult to express your emotions to other people?

___

What happens when you keep your emotions bottled up?

___

What are the positive effects of expressing emotions to others? Any negative effects?

___

How can expressing your emotions improve your emotional well-being?

___

How can expressing your emotions help you get what you want in life?

___

EMOTIONAL WELL-BEING

IDENTIFY and EXPRESS EMOTIONS

Step 3: Keep a Journal of My Emotions

It is important to keep track of the emotions you have a difficult time expressing. Using this page, identify all of the emotions (positive or negative) that you have trouble expressing, to whom, and why it is so difficult to express these emotions.

Emotions I Have Trouble Expressing	To Whom I Have Trouble Expressing Them	Why these Emotions Are Difficult
Love	My wife and children	I assume that they know how I feel, so I don't tell them. My parents didn't tell me, either.

What did you learn about your ability to express emotions to others?

_____

_____

_____

EMOTIONAL WELL-BEING

IDENTIFY and EXPRESS EMOTIONS

Step 4: Set Goals

A well-conceived action plan will help to motivate you as you progress in developing effective skills in expressing your emotions. For this activity, identify goals you have in becoming an effective communicator of your emotions.

The behavior I want to change is _____

Goals need to be SMART:
Specific, **M**easureable, **A**ttainable, **R**ealistic and **T**ime-Specific

Goals	How I Will Measure This Goal	How Is This Goal Attainable and Realistic?	Time Deadline	How This Will Help Me
To tell my spouse how his drinking makes me feel	The number of times I can express my emotions	I can if I have the courage to calmly say how I feel.	By next week-end	I can release my pent-up emotions and maybe he can understand better how and what I'm feeling.

If you are having trouble identifying goals, consult TIPS, page 44.

EMOTIONAL WELL-BEING

IDENTIFY and EXPRESS EMOTIONS

Step 5: Monitor My Behavior – Awareness

You will become a better communicator and be able to express your emotions more effectively if you are in touch with your emotions and be able to truly understand them. Stuffing, ignoring or expressing the wrong emotion will lead to misunderstandings and arguments. Periodic re-evaluations support your success in expressing your emotions well. Once you reach your goal(s), set new ones to improve or maintain what you have already achieved. Use a separate page for each change.

EXAMPLE:

My healthy behavior change   *Interpreting my emotions effectively*

My goal   *To be able to interpret primary and secondary emotions*

Date	My Accomplishment	How It Felt
1/1/2014	I first thought, "What AM I feeling?" and then I told her how I felt.	I felt satisfied because she understood.

✂ -

Awareness

My healthy behavior change _____

My goal _____

Date	My Accomplishment	How It Felt

(Continued on the next page)

EMOTIONAL WELL-BEING

IDENTIFY and EXPRESS EMOTIONS

Step 5: Monitor My Behavior – Body Language

Effective use of body language can help you to be more effective in expressing your emotions. Monitoring your progress toward your body language goals can enhance your progress. Keeping track of your body-language behaviors through logs will help you determine what you have accomplished and what you need to continue working on. Periodic re-evaluations support your success, improve or maintain what you have already achieved and motivate you. Use a separate page for each change.

EXAMPLE:

My healthy behavior change Become more aware of the messages my body sends

My goal Become a student of my own and others' body language

Date	My Accomplishment	How It Felt
1/1/2014	I made an effort to have open body language.	I felt empowered.

Body Language

My healthy behavior change _____

My goal _____

Date	My Accomplishment	How It Felt

(Continued on the next page)

EMOTIONAL WELL-BEING

IDENTIFY and EXPRESS EMOTIONS

Step 5: Monitor My Behavior – Direct

Effective communication is direct communication, and this is especially true when expressing your emotions. Use the following chart to monitor your progress toward your goals, reinforce your behavior, and determine what you have accomplished at given times. Periodic re-evaluations will help you create new communication goals. Once you reach your goal(s), set new ones to improve or maintain what you have already achieved. Use a separate page for each change.

EXAMPLE:

My healthy behavior change Communicate my emotions without anger or a loud voice

My goal To express my emotions to my son

Date	My Accomplishment	How It Felt
1/1/2014	I calmly told my son how anxious I become when he stays out late and how much I worry.	I felt a connection with him that was not there before.

Direct

My healthy behavior change _____

My goal _____

Date	My Accomplishment	How It Felt

EMOTIONAL WELL-BEING

IDENTIFY and EXPRESS EMOTIONS

Step 6: Reward Myself

When you express your emotions well to someone, you need to reward yourself! For most people, it can be awkward to reward yourself. Regardless, you will find that you are more likely to repeat behaviors if you do find a way to give yourself a reward. Your reward should give you the incentive to achieve your goals, be within your budget and be something you'll be excited about. If you are buying yourself something, be sure your reward is something you wouldn't ordinarily buy or do.

- Rewards that would be meaningful to me _____
- Small rewards I could give myself _____
- Large rewards I could give myself _____
- Things that would not cost money and would be fun _____
- Rewards that I can afford and that would be fun _____
- Rewards that I enjoy alone _____
- Rewards I enjoy with people who support me _____

You deserve a pat on the back for the hard work you are completing in this session. Rewards help you to pay attention to your triumphs, not your setbacks. Rewards will create good feelings and propel you to want to work harder to reach your goals. Whenever you have completed or achieved one of your goals, treat yourself to one of the items on your list. You can also reward yourself by giving yourself positive affirmations when you have achieved a goal. Below are some samples. Cut them out and post in visible spots at home and work! If these don't work for your goal, write your own on sticky notes!

It feels good to express my emotions!	Keeping emotions bottled up is not good for me!	I can be direct without raising my voice.
I can be open, honest and direct.	I am aware of other people's body language.	I am a better communicator!
It is becoming easier to say what I want.	When I want to express how I feel, I will start my sentences with "I feel."	*I am aware of my own body language.*

"If you don't manage your emotions, then your emotions will manage you!"

~ **Doc Childre and Deborah Rozman**

EMOTIONAL WELL-BEING

IDENTIFY and EXPRESS EMOTIONS

Step 7: Tips for Motivated Behavior Modification

Awareness

- Be honest with yourself about what you are feeling. Don't let others tell you how you are feeling.
- Remember that anger can obscure other emotions such as jealousy, sadness, fear, loneliness and disappointment.
- Trust your feelings.
- Keep a *Feelings Journal* to become more aware of your feelings in general.
- Remember that tuning into your emotions, especially negative ones like anger, sadness and jealousy, can be painful to experience; it is natural tendency is to repress them. This allows you to feel better at the time, but pent-up emotions can fester and cause problems later on.

Body Language

- Notice others body language behaviors including tone of voice, facial expressions, movements, posture, eye content, speech patterns, reactions and gestures.
- Remember that a person's body language is based on signals that are not consciously chosen.
- Attempt to pick up on body language signals that may be communicating information to you.
- Behavior often speaks louder than your words.
- Eighty percent of all communication is accomplished through body language.

Direct

- Get to the main idea of what you want to convey to the other person.
- Express your emotions in an assertive (honest, open and direct) way and then support them with explanations.
- Make a point to ask listeners if they understand the points and emotions you are trying to convey.
- Express your emotions rather than venting your emotions
- Express facts. If you express opinions, say so, and be open to others' opinions.
- Express your emotions in a normal tone and volume.
- Express your emotions directly by using statements such as "When you told me that last night, I felt _____ ."

SECTION III
BALANCE WORK and PERSONAL LIFE

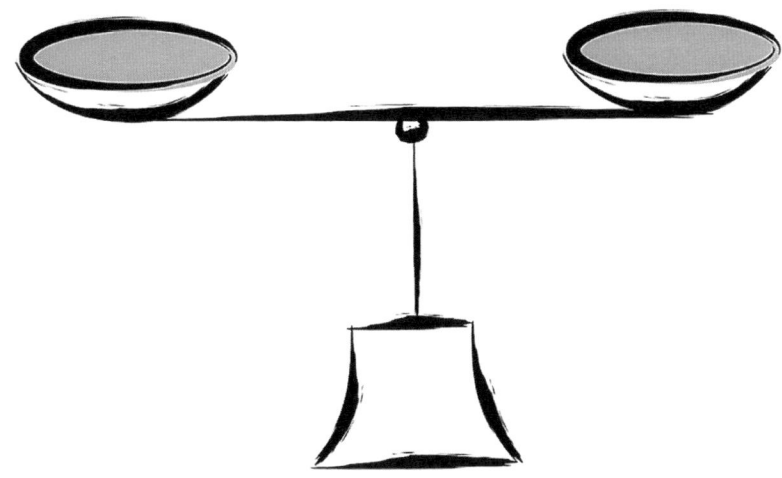

"A time for work and a time for play – balance in all things."

~ Jonathan Lockwood Huie

Name _____

Date _____

EMOTIONAL WELL-BEING

EMOTIONAL WELL-BEING

BALANCE WORK and PERSONAL LIFE

Step 1: Self-Assessment Introduction and Directions

Many people today find it challenging to juggle the demands of their work life and the demands of their personal life. The combination of work deadlines and required extra hours, combined with increased family responsibilities, can make balance in life very difficult to achieve.

This self-assessment contains 30 statements related to your effectiveness in balancing your work and personal life. Read each item carefully and decide how much the statement describes you. In each of the choices listed, circle the number of your response.

In the following example, the circled number 2 indicates the statement is True for the person completing the inventory.

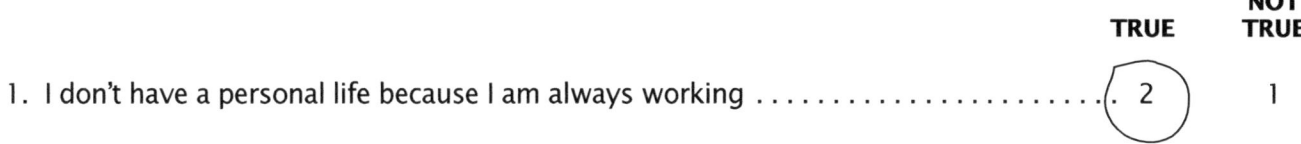

	TRUE	NOT TRUE
1. I don't have a personal life because I am always working	(2)	1

This is not a test and there are no right or wrong answers. Do not spend too much time thinking about your answers. Your initial response will be the most true for you. Be sure to respond to every statement.

Turn the page and complete the Self-Assessment

EMOTIONAL WELL-BEING

BALANCE WORK and PERSONAL LIFE

Step 1: Self-Assessment

	TRUE	NOT TRUE
1. I don't have a personal life because I am always working	2	1
2. My job consumes too much of my time as it is	1	2
3. I rarely bring work home with me	1	2
4. I often feel I must drop everything else for my work	2	1
5. I have lots of hobbies	1	2
6. I feel like I can never finish my work	2	1
7. I do not think ahead or set goals at work	1	2
8. Personal time is just time off to rest up for the next workday	2	1
9. I feel guilty if I'm having too much fun	2	1
10. I often do work-related jobs in my spare time	2	1
11. I am able to juggle the demands of my job and my personal life	1	2
12. I judge myself by my accomplishments at work	2	1
13. I don't have enough time for family and friends	2	1
14. My personal life is as important as the work I do	1	2
15. I try not to take on too many additional tasks at work	1	2
16. I am more interested in my work than my personal life	2	1
17. I rarely obsess over work to be done	1	2
18. I usually work more than eight hours per day	2	1
19. I rarely work evenings and weekends	1	2
20. I "escape" from the house, chores and family by going to work	2	1
21. I am often unable to relax after work	2	1
22. I am constantly thinking about work	2	1
23. I feel guilty when I'm not working	2	1
24. I can't wait for my next vacation	1	2
25. I often spend my free time in activities not related to work	1	2
26. I get bored when I am not working	2	1
27. I go to work even if I'm sick	2	1
28. I cope with life's problems by working harder	2	1
29. I put in lots of extra hours working	2	1
30. I do not know how to spend my time off	2	1

Total = _____

Go to the Scoring Directions on the next page

EMOTIONAL WELL-BEING

BALANCE WORK and PERSONAL LIFE

Step 1: Self-Assessment Scoring Directions

The *Balance Work and Personal Life Self-Assessment* is designed to help you identify how you balance your personal and work or volunteer life. On the self-assessment page, add the numbers that you circled in each section and write the scores on each of the TOTAL lines. You will receive a total in the range from 30 to 60. Then, transfer those numbers to the space below.

Work-Life Balance Total = _____

Profile Interpretation

Individual Score	Result	Indications
30 to 39	Low	If you scored in this range, your work and personal life are out of balance. You need to develop a few healthier work-life balance habits.
40 to 50	Moderate	If you scored in this range, your work and personal life are somewhat out of balance. You need to develop some healthier work-life balance habits.
51 to 60	High	If you scored in this range, your work and personal life are extremely out of balance. You need to develop many healthier work-life balance habits.

Step 1: Self-Assessment Description

Balancing Work and Personal Life is critical in maintaining your emotional well-being. People who score high on this scale tend to be workaholics and often ignore their personal lives. They derive their primary identity from the work they do and seem to be happiest while in the workplace. They will work extra hours and bring work home in the evenings and weekends if they have to. They like to work in their spare time and tend to get bored when not working. They do not have many leisure time activities and often do not enjoy the ones they have. Their work tends to be more important and satisfying than their personal lives.

EMOTIONAL WELL-BEING

BALANCE WORK and PERSONAL LIFE

Step 2: Recognize and Develop a Support System

Balancing your work and personal life takes support from friends, family and people in the community. To have a more balanced approach to life, you need the support of people you know who can help. Not every supportive person in your life will be helpful with this, but some will. Complete the following table with people who might be able to support you with your efforts to balance your personal and work life.

Supporter	How This Person Can Support Me	How I Can Contact This Person
My friend James	He is a good worker and manages to have time for family and friends, too.	phone or text: 000-0001 email: james22@.com

Keep this list handy. Call, email or text when you need support.

EMOTIONAL WELL-BEING

BALANCE WORK and PERSONAL LIFE

Step 3: Keep a Journal

Journaling is an excellent way for you to truly look at your behaviors related to balancing your work, volunteer and personal life. The questions that follow have been designed to help you think with an open mind about your current behaviors. Remember, your thinking can affect how motivated you are to make sincere changes in the amounts of time you are spending in your work and/or volunteer life and personal life.

What in your life is out of balance? _____
_____
_____

How can you use your time more effectively? _____
_____
_____

How can you begin spending personal, volunteer and work time, each in a reasonable amount? _____
_____
_____

How does imbalance between your work and personal life cause stress to you personally? _____
_____
_____

How does it cause stress between you and your family? _____
_____
_____

How does it cause stress between you and your friends? _____
_____
_____

How does it cause stress between you and your work or volunteer place? _____
_____
_____

How can you better control the number of hours you put in at work, volunteer and personal time? ___
_____
_____

EMOTIONAL WELL-BEING

BALANCE WORK and PERSONAL LIFE

Step 4: Set Goals

Action planning is an important step in achieving lasting behavioral changes. Action planning will ensure you remain motivated in your efforts to balance your work and personal life. For your action plan, identify both the specific behaviors you want to change, and develop goals and smaller goals required to reach your ultimate work, volunteer and personal life balance goals.

The behavior I want to change is _____

Goals need to be SMART:
Specific, **M**easureable, **A**ttainable, **R**ealistic and **T**ime-Specific

Goals	How I Will Measure This Goal	How Is This Goal Attainable and Realistic?	Time Deadline	How This Will Help Me
Work a 40-hour workweek	Keep track of the number of hours I work	Yes, eventually I will be able to maintain a standard schedule.	By the end of next month	I will have more time to work on my relationships.

If you are having trouble identifying goals, consult TIPS, page 58.

EMOTIONAL WELL-BEING

BALANCE WORK and PERSONAL LIFE

Step 5: Monitor My Behavior – Work Life

Maintaining balance between your work and personal life requires you to monitor how much time you are spending, or not spending, on a job. The following chart will help you keep track of your work life goals. Identify some work life goals and then periodically re-evaluate them. Once you reach your work life goal(s), set new ones to improve or maintain what you have already achieved. Use a separate page for each change.

EXAMPLE:

My healthy behavior change Work smarter, not longer

My goal Manage my time better on the job so I get more done

Date	My Accomplishment	How It Felt
1/1/2014	I didn't talk so much with my co-workers.	I was happy to have more time to myself.

Work Life

My healthy behavior change_____

My goal _____

Date	My Accomplishment	How It Felt

(Continued on the next page)

EMOTIONAL WELL-BEING

BALANCE WORK and PERSONAL LIFE

Step 5: Monitor My Behavior – Work Life (Continued)

Complete the following table to explore time-management problems that might be keeping you at work longer and hindering you from getting your work done on time.

Time Management Problems at Work	How I can Manage My Work Time Better	How I Can Have More Time After Work

How will managing your time more effectively help you achieve greater balance between your work and personal life?

_____

_____

EMOTIONAL WELL-BEING

BALANCE WORK and PERSONAL LIFE

Step 5: Monitor My Behavior – Personal Life

Maintaining balance between your work and personal life requires you to also monitor how much time you are spending, or not spending, on developing a personal life outside of work. Think about, write down, and then monitor your goals for your personal life. Don't forget to periodically re-evaluate them and once you reach your personal life goal(s), set new ones to improve or maintain what you have already achieved. Use a separate page for each change.

EXAMPLE:

My healthy behavior change Stop my multi-tasking and listen more effectively

My goal Develop a "Things-To-Do" list and concentrate on one at a time

Date	My Accomplishment	How It Felt
1/1/2014	I listened attentively to my daughter about school without doing anything else.	It felt good to focus on the conversation without being distracted.

Personal Life

My healthy behavior change _____

My goal _____

Date	My Accomplishment	How It Felt

(Continued on the next page)

EMOTIONAL WELL-BEING

BALANCE WORK and PERSONAL LIFE

Step 5: Monitor My Behavior – Personal Life *(Continued)*

What are your consistent time management issues? (home, work, family, community, etc.)

_____
_____
_____

How are you affected by your time management issues?

_____
_____
_____

How are others in your life affected by your time management issues?

_____
_____
_____

What obstacles do you envision in adopting new time-management behaviors?

_____
_____
_____

What will you gain by adopting new time-management behaviors?

_____
_____
_____

What will people close to you gain by your adopting new time-management behaviors?

_____
_____
_____

EMOTIONAL WELL-BEING

BALANCE WORK and PERSONAL LIFE

Step 6: Reward Myself

In society today, it can be difficult to balance your work and personal life, and when you do you deserve a reward! But what type of reward would keep you motivated? The answer to this question will be different for each person. Your reward needs to be something that will give you the incentive to achieve your goals. It needs to be within your budget and something you'll be excited about. If you are buying yourself something, be sure your reward is something you wouldn't ordinarily buy or do. Remember that some of the best things in life are free.

- Rewards that would be meaningful to me _____
- Small rewards I could give myself _____
- Large rewards I could give myself _____
- Things that would not cost money and would be fun _____
- Rewards that I can afford and that would be fun _____
- Rewards that I enjoy alone _____
- Rewards I enjoy with people who support me _____

You deserve a pat on the back for the hard work you are completing in this session. Rewards help you to pay attention to your triumphs, not your setbacks. Rewards will create good feelings and propel you to want to work harder to reach your goals. Whenever you have completed or achieved one of your goals, treat yourself to one of the items on your list. You can also reward yourself by giving yourself positive affirmations when you have achieved a goal. Below are some samples. Cut them out and post in visible spots at home and work! If these don't work for your goal, write your own on sticky notes!

I enjoy it when my lifestyle is well-balanced.	I am productive in all areas of my life.	I am using my time wisely.
Work-Life balance is critical!	I will limit the work I bring home!	I'm not as stressed when I'm not working so much.
I control how I spend my time.	I am creating a harmonious life.	*All of my goals are in balance.*

Hillary Clinton urged us, "Don't confuse having a career with having a life." How do you confuse the two?

_____

_____

EMOTIONAL WELL-BEING

BALANCE WORK and PERSONAL LIFE

Step 7: Tips for Motivated Behavior Modification

Work Life

- Stop behaviors that take up too much of your time and energy. For example, walking around and visiting with your co-workers might be keeping you from getting your work done in a timely way.

- Stay focused and prioritize your tasks and goals.

- Organize. Discipline yourself to work on the most important tasks you have to complete.

- Manage your time efficiently. Eliminate any activities that are unimportant. Improve your planning skills so that you are using your time at work efficiently.

- Minimize the work you bring home on the weekends and evenings. If you can, delegate your duties or train other employees to cover responsibilities when you are away from work.

- Limit distractions at work that keep you from doing your job.

Personal Life

- Schedule yourself some time during the week to spend with family, friends, or your favorite leisure activities.

- Make time during the week for regular exercise. Exercising is an excellent way to engage in physical activity. Aerobic exercises, running, jogging and walking release endorphins that help reduce stress.

- Create and maintain a support system with people outside of work. These people can help to recharge you after challenging times.

- Spend time each week doing things you enjoy that are frivolous and help take your mind off of your work. These activities might include going to the park, talking with friends, or playing a game with family members.

SECTION IV
MAINTAIN a HOPEFUL OUTLOOK

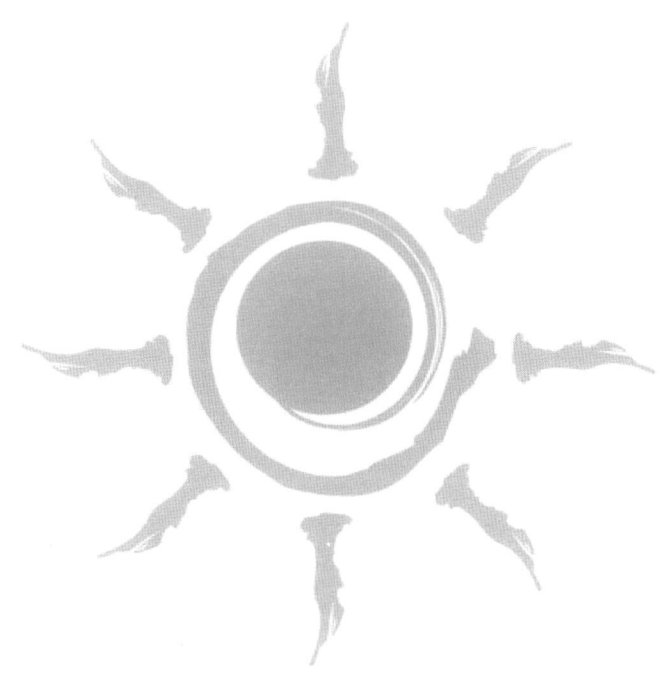

"A pessimist sees the difficulty in every opportunity; an optimist sees the opportunity in every difficulty."

~ Winston Churchill

Name _____

Date _____

EMOTIONAL WELL-BEING

EMOTIONAL WELL-BEING

MAINTAIN a HOPEFUL OUTLOOK

Step 1: Self-Assessment Introduction and Directions

Some people see the glass half full, while others see it half empty. The people who see the glass half full are optimists, and they tend to be able to maintain a hopeful outlook regardless of what is happening in their lives. When they encounter setbacks or disappointments optimists look at the bright side and see the possibilities in what is happening in their lives. They anticipate good things will happen, expect to be able to solve problems efficiently, and plan to accomplish their life and work goals. They go through life with a positive outlook and are content most of the time.

The *Maintain a Hopeful Outlook Self-Assessment* is designed to help you be aware of your outlook when negative and positive things happen in your life. This scale contains 40 statements that are divided into four resiliency categories. Read each of the statements and decide whether or not the statement describes you. Circle the number of your response on the line to the right of each statement.

In the following example, the circled 3 indicates the statement is very much like the person completing the assessment:

	VERY MUCH LIKE ME	USUALLY LIKE ME	NOT USUALLY LIKE ME	NOT LIKE ME
1. Even when things go wrong, I remain hopeful	4	3	2	1

This is not a test and there are no right or wrong answers. Do not spend too much time thinking about your answers. Your initial response will be the most true for you. Be sure to respond to every statement.

Turn the page and complete the Self-Assessment

EMOTIONAL WELL-BEING

MAINTAIN a HOPEFUL OUTLOOK

Step 1: Self-Assessment

	VERY MUCH LIKE ME	USUALLY LIKE ME	NOT USUALLY LIKE ME	NOT LIKE ME
1. Even when things go wrong, I remain hopeful	4	3	2	1
2. My difficult situations do not have positive outcomes	1	2	3	4
3. I can see the positive in most situations	4	3	2	1
4. I often feel like my life is hopeless.	1	2	3	4
5. I look on the bright side of things.	4	3	2	1
6. I am optimistic about my future	4	3	2	1
7. I am unhappy a lot of the time.	1	2	3	4
8. My self-thoughts are positive.	4	3	2	1
9. I look for situations that keep me feeling good.	4	3	2	1
10. I feel helpless when things in my life change	1	2	3	4

H – TOTAL = _____

11. When things in my life change, I expect the best	4	3	2	1
12. If anything can go wrong in my life, it probably will	1	2	3	4
13. I expect things to go my way	4	3	2	1
14. Things don't work out the way I want them to	1	2	3	4
15. I am afraid to hope that good things will happen to me	1	2	3	4
16. I wonder why good things never happen to me	1	2	3	4
17. My problems never seem to end.	1	2	3	4
18. Even though I have failed in the past, I do not expect to fail again	4	3	2	1
19. I maintain a positive attitude in life.	4	3	2	1
20. I feel like I have no control over what happens in my life	1	2	3	4

L – TOTAL = _____

Continued on the next page

EMOTIONAL WELL-BEING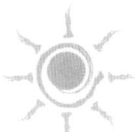

MAINTAIN a HOPEFUL OUTLOOK

Step 1: Self-Assessment *(continued)*

	VERY MUCH LIKE ME	USUALLY LIKE ME	NOT USUALLY LIKE ME	NOT LIKE ME
21. I talk about positive things.	4	3	2	1
22. I do not see good things in people	1	2	3	4
23. I see the positive side of situations, not the negative	4	3	2	1
24. I have a hard time seeing the possibilities in a situation	1	2	3	4
25. Every day holds many opportunities.	4	3	2	1
26. When faced with a challenge, my first thought is hopeful curiosity.	4	3	2	1
27. I remain positive even when things do not go my way.	4	3	2	1
28. Each day presents new opportunities for success and happiness.	4	3	2	1
29. I find myself waiting for happiness to find me.	1	2	3	4
30. I believe that things will work out the way I want.	4	3	2	1

A – TOTAL = _____

31. I set specific life goals and work toward them	4	3	2	1
32. I lack confidence in myself.	1	2	3	4
33. I believe I can do whatever I set my mind to.	4	3	2	1
34. I will not quit at the first sign of a problem.	4	3	2	1
35. I will take calculated chances even if it doesn't work out	4	3	2	1
36. I blame my misfortunes on others.	1	2	3	4
37. I do not let obstacles get in my way.	4	3	2	1
38. I do not blame others when bad things happen to me	4	3	2	1
39. When people say "it's impossible," I believe them	1	2	3	4
40. I allow myself to let others keep me from being hopeful	1	2	3	4

O – TOTAL = _____

Go to the Scoring Directions on the next page

EMOTIONAL WELL-BEING

MAINTAIN a HOPEFUL OUTLOOK

Step 1: Self Assessment Scoring Directions

Resilient people are able to maintain a positive outlook in life. They are able to remain hopeful about their current situations and future possibilities, expect good things to happen from their efforts, and retain a positive attitude even when life is challenging. Resilient people work hard to overcome obstacles. For each of the four sections on the previous pages, total the scores you circled. Put that total on the line marked TOTAL at the end of each section.

Then, transfer your totals to the spaces below:

H – HOPE   TOTAL = _____

L – LIFE OUTLOOK   TOTAL = _____

A – ATTITUDE   TOTAL = _____

O – OVERCOMING OBSTACLES TOTAL = _____

Profile Interpretation

Individual Scales Scores	Total Scales Scores	Result	Indications
Scores from 31 to 40	Scores from 121 to 160	High	You have many skills and attitudes that lead to a positive outlook and a resilient personality.
Scores from 20 to 30	Scores from 81 to 120	Moderate	You have some skills and attitudes that lead to a positive outlook and a resilient personality.
Scores from 10 to 19	Scores from 40 to 80	Low	You do not have enough skills and attitudes that will lead to positive outlooks and a resilient personality.

For scales scored in the moderate or low range, find the descriptions on the pages that follow. Read the description and complete the exercises that are included. No matter how you scored, low, moderate or high, you will benefit from these exercises.

EMOTIONAL WELL-BEING

MAINTAIN a HOPEFUL OUTLOOK

Step 1: Self-Assessment Descriptions

H – HOPE – People scoring high on this scale are able to remain hopeful regardless of the situation in which they find themselves. They always try to look at the bright side of things and remain optimistic and hopeful about their future.

L – LIFE OUTLOOK – People scoring high on this scale expect the best regardless of the situation in which they find themselves. They believe that life, even difficult situations, presents opportunities. They actively seek out those opportunities.

A – ATTITUDE – People scoring high on this scale have a positive attitude regardless of the situation in which they find themselves. They look for the good in each situation and each person, and they believe that things will work out the way they want.

O – OVERCOMING OBSTACLES – People scoring high on this scale don't let obstacles get in their way regardless of the situation in which they find themselves. They take responsibility for their lives and do not blame others. They also believe they can succeed regardless of what others say.

Step 2: Recognize and Develop a Support System

Maintaining a hopeful outlook can be challenging and you need people to talk to when you become less than optimistic. Complete the following table with people who might be able to support you in developing and maintaining hopeful emotions and a hopeful outlook.

Supporter	How This Person Can Support Me	How I Can Contact This Person
My father	By continually reminding me that good things are on the horizon	phone 000-000-0000

Keep this list handy. Call, email or text when you need support.

EMOTIONAL WELL-BEING

MAINTAIN a HOPEFUL OUTLOOK

Step 3: Keep a Journal

Journaling is the practice of exploring your emotions about the events in your life. These journaling items will help you to explore how well you have been at maintaining a hopeful outlook in your life. Please complete the following items so that you can better understand your outlook and its effect on your life.

In what ways are you optimistic about your future?

_____
_____
_____

How would you describe your attitude about life? How can you make it even more positive?

_____
_____
_____

How has failure in the past stopped you from taking chances?

_____
_____
_____

What types of things do you worry about from your past?

_____
_____
_____

What people or events zap you of energy?

_____
_____
_____

What are you passionate about?

_____
_____
_____

EMOTIONAL WELL-BEING

MAINTAIN a HOPEFUL OUTLOOK

Step 4: Set Goals

Hope is one of the greatest emotions that you can possess. When people are hopeful, they believe that they can do anything. To develop a hopeful attitude, you need to develop hope-related goals. These are goals that you can work toward, and when completed, will motivate you to do more! For your action plan below, identify ways that you can be more hopeful and maintain a positive outlook about your life.

The behavior I want to change is _____

Goals need to be SMART:
Specific, Measureable, Attainable, Realistic and Time-Specific

Goals	How I Will Measure This Goal	How Is This Goal Attainable and Realistic?	Time Deadline	How This Will Help Me
I want to be more optimistic.	How often I am optimistic about my future	I can work on it and make it happen.	End of summer	I will feel so much more content.

If you are having trouble identifying goals, consult TIPS, page 73.

EMOTIONAL WELL-BEING

MAINTAIN a HOPEFUL OUTLOOK

Step 5: Monitor My Behavior – Hope

Hope is a tremendous emotion to possess. When you are hopeful, you believe all things are possible. Setting hope-related goals and monitoring your progress toward those goals will help to reinforce a hopeful outlook about life. The following chart will guide you through the development and tracking of hopeful outlook goals. Review your behaviors periodically to ensure you are progressing in your pursuit of a hopeful outlook. Once you reach a goal, set new ones to continue to develop hope in your life. Use a separate page for each change.

EXAMPLE:

My healthy behavior change   I need to stop complaining so much.

My goal   I want people to want to be with me.

Date	My Accomplishment	How It Felt
1/1/2014	I did not complain once today.	Hopeful. I'll keep going.

Hope

My healthy behavior change _____

My goal _____

Date	My Accomplishment	How It Felt

(Continued on the next page)

EMOTIONAL WELL-BEING

MAINTAIN a HOPEFUL OUTLOOK

Step 5: Monitor My Behavior – Life Outlook

Do you always see the glass half-empty? If so you are not alone, but it is time to begin to see the glass half-full! Use the chart that follows to set some goals to work toward that will help you improve your life outlook. Keep track of your progress by monitoring your behavior, to help you determine how successful you have been in developing a positive life outlook. Once you reach your goal(s) related to your life outlook, set new ones to improve or maintain what you have already achieved. Use a separate page for each change.

EXAMPLE:

My healthy behavior change *I need to stop worrying about the past.*

My goal *To accept that I made mistakes in the past, get over them and move on.*

Date	My Accomplishment	How It Felt
1/1/2014	I was able to stay in the present most of the day.	Wonderful

✂ -

Life Outlook

My healthy behavior change _____

My goal _____

Date	My Accomplishment	How It Felt

(Continued on the next page)

EMOTIONAL WELL-BEING

MAINTAIN a HOPEFUL OUTLOOK

Step 5: Monitor My Behavior – Attitude

A positive emotional attitude will serve you well in your personal and professional life. In the spaces that follow, identify some of the goals you have for enhancing your attitude about life. These goals should be related to seeing opportunities, believing everything will work out well and looking at the positive side. Monitoring your progress toward these types of goals will help you develop a more positive attitude. Keep track of your behaviors through the logs, re-evaluate your success, then set new goals to enhance what you have already achieved. Use a separate page for each change.

EXAMPLE:

My healthy behavior change   *I must eliminate my negative thinking.*
My goal   *To maintain a positive attitude about my spouse working late*

Date	My Accomplishment	How It Felt
1/1/2014	Every time a negative thought popped into my head, I just said "Stop!"	Liberating

✂ --

Attitude

My healthy behavior change _____

My goal _____

Date	My Accomplishment	How It Felt

(Continued on the next page)

EMOTIONAL WELL-BEING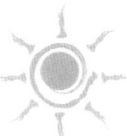

MAINTAIN a HOPEFUL OUTLOOK

Step 5: Monitor My Behavior – Overcoming Obstacles

All people face obstacles, but the truly successful people in life are able to find ways to overcome these obstacles. You can too! To get started, use the space below to set some goals for overcoming obstacles, monitoring your progress toward your goals, and keep track of your behaviors through logs. Periodic re-evaluations support your success. Once you reach a goal that will help you overcome obstacles, set new ones to improve or maintain what you have already achieved. Use a separate page for each change.

EXAMPLE:

My healthy behavior change   I want to stop blaming my situation on other people.
My goal   To take more responsibility for my present life and my future life

Date	My Accomplishment	How It Felt
1/1/2014	I stopped blaming my mother for my lack of education and enrolled in the local college.	It felt good to overcome my education obstacle. This will influence my future outlook.

Overcoming Obstacles

My healthy behavior change_____

My goal_____

Date	My Accomplishment	How It Felt

EMOTIONAL WELL-BEING

MAINTAIN a HOPEFUL OUTLOOK

Step 6: Reward Myself

Hope is the feeling or emotion that everything will turn out okay or that you can succeed or get what you want. Hope is a positive emotion that helps you to keep going forward even in times of adversity. As you complete goals and find yourself becoming more hopeful, you need to reward yourself. These rewards need to be something that will give you the incentive to achieve even more goals. It needs to be within your budget and something you'll be excited about. If you are buying yourself something, be sure your reward is something you wouldn't ordinarily buy or do. Brainstorm possible rewards.

- Rewards that would be meaningful to me _____
- Small rewards I could give myself _____
- Large rewards I could give myself _____
- Things that would not cost money and would be fun _____
- Rewards that I can afford and that would be fun _____
- Rewards that I enjoy alone _____
- Rewards I enjoy with people who support me _____

You deserve a pat on the back for the hard work you are completing in this chapter. Rewards help you to pay attention to your triumphs, not your setbacks. Rewards will create good feelings and propel you to want to work harder to reach your goals. Whenever you have completed or achieved one of your goals, treat yourself to one of the items on your list. You can also reward yourself by giving yourself positive affirmations when you have achieved a goal. Below are some samples. Cut them out and post in visible spots at home and work! If these don't work for your goal, write your own on sticky notes!

I can make good things happen.	Today will be an awesome day.	I see opportunities everywhere!
I love ME!	I choose optimistic thoughts.	I have faith in myself.
Each day I feel more positive about myself.	I expect things to go my way.	*I am excited to see what today brings!*

"Once you replace negative thoughts with positive ones, you'll start having positive results."

~ Willie Nelson

EMOTIONAL WELL-BEING

MAINTAIN a HOPEFUL OUTLOOK

Step 7: Tips for Motivated Behavior Modification

Hope
- Remain hopeful and try to see the positives in any situation.
- Visualize positive things happening in your life.
- Intentionally engage in activities that you find enjoyable.
- Stop complaining and start building the future you deserve.
- Don't allow people or things to drain your energy.
- Follow your passions.

Life Outlook
- Stay in the present.
- Do not worry about the past or fixate too much on the future.
- Be with people who are positive, who uplift you, and who keep you focused on the positive aspects of your life.
- Expect the best from yourself.
- All people have problems – learn to overcome yours.

Attitude
- Look for opportunities everywhere you go and in everything you do.
- Sometimes life gets so frantic that it is easy to become negative. Negative expectations will trigger negative emotions and eliminate positive ones.
- By staying mindful on the positive, you can let go of negative thoughts and begin to experience more positive ones.
- Often times when you hear your negative inner voice, it is not your own thoughts. It is often the voices of other people who have spoken to you in past times and these thoughts have stayed with you.
- Believe in yourself and soon others will believe in you.

Overcoming Obstacles
- Take calculated risks when necessary.
- Most people have failed in some way in their past. Failure is nothing to be ashamed of, as long as you don't dwell on your failures, but learn from them and go forward.
- What have you learned from your failures?
- Have you grown from your failures?
- Have confidence in your ability to overcome obstacles and enhance your self-confidence.

EMOTIONAL WELL-BEING

SECTION V

FEEL GOOD ABOUT YOURSELF

"You really have to look inside yourself and find your own inner strength and say, 'I'm proud of what I am and who I am, and I'm just going to be myself.'"

~ Mariah Carey

Name _____

Date _____

EMOTIONAL WELL-BEING

EMOTIONAL WELL-BEING

FEEL GOOD ABOUT YOURSELF

Step 1: Self-Assessment Introduction and Directions

Feeling good about yourself is critical in living a satisfying life. Self-esteem refers to the notion that you are an important and valuable person because of who you are. People with high self-esteem feel they are worthy and as valuable as anyone else. They are happy to be who they are and respect themselves. The *Feel Good About Yourself* Self-Assessment will help you explore your levels of self-esteem as it is related to your overall emotional wellness.

This assessment contains 28 statements related to your self-worth. Read each of the statements and decide whether or not the statement describes you. If the statement *does* describe you, circle the number in the YES column. If the statement *does not* describe you, circle the number in the NO column.

In the following example, the circled number under YES indicates the statement is descriptive of the person completing the inventory.

	YES	NO
I constantly criticize myself...	(1)	2

This is not a test and there are no right or wrong answers. Do not spend too much time thinking about your answers. Your initial response will be the most true for you. Be sure to respond to every statement.

Turn the page and complete the Self-Assessment

EMOTIONAL WELL-BEING

FEEL GOOD ABOUT YOURSELF

Step 1: Self-Assessment

	YES	NO
I constantly criticize myself	1	2
I have many positive skills and qualities	2	1
I accept the fact that I'm not perfect	2	1
I have special talents	2	1
I understand how I am special	2	1
I have a difficult time accepting and liking myself	1	2
I often compare myself to others with envy	1	2

P – TOTAL _____

I usually do what I think is right	2	1
I often exaggerate the truth to maintain my image	1	2
I am content with what I have and who I am	2	1
I often feel ashamed of myself	1	2
I make excuses when I make mistakes	1	2
I talk about my accomplishments	2	1
I would not change much about myself	2	1

I – TOTAL _____

(Continued on the next page)

EMOTIONAL WELL-BEING

FEEL GOOD ABOUT YOURSELF

Step 1: Self-Assessment *(Continued)*

	YES	NO
I usually see the glass half full	2	1
I worry about things beyond my control	1	2
I usually look at the bright side of things	2	1
I am not a very positive person	1	2
My first reaction is I can't or it can't be done	1	2
I relive my mistakes over and over	1	2
I see success in my future	2	1

O – TOTAL _____

	YES	NO
I worry excessively about what other people say about me	1	2
I feel rejected when others pay little attention to me	1	2
I compare myself favorably to others	2	1
My personal self-worth is related to others' opinions of me	1	2
I don't need all people to like and accept me	2	1
I'm not sure I've done a good job until someone tells me so.	1	2
My own opinions count more to me than others' opinions	2	1

S – TOTAL _____

Go to the Scoring Directions on the next page

EMOTIONAL WELL-BEING

FEEL GOOD ABOUT YOURSELF

Step 1: Self Assessment Scoring Directions

Self-esteem is how you feel about yourself. It is your perception of your worth, as well as your perception of what others think of you. Good self-esteem is being able to think and speak positively and confidently about yourself without bragging or being arrogant. It is critical in your emotional well-being and your overall happiness in life.

The *Feel Good About Yourself* Self-Assessment is designed to help you explore various aspects of your perceived self-esteem. On the previous two pages, add the numbers that you circled in each section and write the scores on each of the TOTAL lines. You will receive a total in the range from 7 to 14. The, transfer those numbers to the spaces below.

P = Pride   Total = _____

I = Image   Total = _____

O = Outlook   Total = _____

S = Self-Approval Total = _____

Profile Interpretation

Individual Scale Score	Result	Indications
7 to 9	Low	You have a limited perceived belief in your own self-esteem. It is important for you to develop a better image of yourself, be aware of your positive traits, accept yourself as you are, and who you can become, maintain a positive view of life, and not overly rely on the opinions of others.
10 to 11	Moderate	You have a fairly healthy belief in your own self-esteem. It is important for you to develop an even better image of yourself, be aware of your positive traits, accept yourself as you are, and who you can become, maintain a positive view of life, and not overly rely on the opinions of others.
12 to 14	High	You have a very healthy belief in your own self-esteem. It is important for you to continue to develop your image of yourself, be aware of your positive traits, accept yourself as you are, and who you can become, maintain a positive view of life, and not overly rely on the opinions of others.

No matter how you scored on the Scale (Low, Moderate or High), you will benefit from doing all of the following exercises.

EMOTIONAL WELL-BEING

FEEL GOOD ABOUT YOURSELF

Step 1: Self-Assessment Descriptions

Pride -- People scoring high on this scale tend to accept themselves for who they are and accept their imperfections as well as their positive qualities. They are proud of themselves and their accomplishments. They have special talents and are not critical of themselves.

Image – People scoring high on this scale feel confident and comfortable with themselves and do not spend time wishing they were different. Their image is related to their character, self-worth and value as a person. They maintain a positive image of themselves.

Outlook – People scoring high on this scale have an outlook on life that is generally upbeat and positive. They see the brighter, optimistic viewpoints, tend not to blame themselves too much, persevere through setbacks and obstacles, and find joy in small things in life. They take the opportunity to learn from their mistakes and look upon them as valuable life lessons.

Self-Approval – People scoring high on this scale do what they believe to be right for them, behave according to their values, and what is right for the greater good. They will listen to the opinions of others and consider their thoughts in their decision making. They do not make value judgments about themselves based on others' opinions. They realize there is no connection between their personal worth and how people feel about them.

Step 2: Recognize and Develop a Support System

There are times when you are unable to recognize your positive qualities and accomplishments. When this happens you need to rely on your support system, or those people who are able to remind you of all of your positive qualities. Complete the following table with people who might help you feel good about yourself.

Supporter	How This Person Can Support Me	How I Can Contact This Person
My Significant Other	He often reminds me of how much I have accomplished in life.	At home or on the phone

Keep this list handy. Call, email or text when you need support.

EMOTIONAL WELL-BEING

FEEL GOOD ABOUT YOURSELF

Step 3: Keep a Journal

Your self-esteem is your overall emotional evaluation of your worth as a human being. Journaling exercises can help you re-evaluate yourself and your worth. The following questions are designed to help you think conscientiously about the self-esteem issues you want to change. Please share your honest thoughts and emotions you have about yourself.

What do you like most about yourself? _____

_____

What do you like least about yourself? _____

_____

Can you change that? How? _____

_____

If you cannot change that; how can you be satisfied to be just as you are? _____

In what ways do you feel good about yourself? _____

_____

In what ways don't you feel good about yourself? _____

_____

Can you change that? How? _____

_____

If you cannot change that; how can you be satisfied to be just as you are? _____

_____

In what ways do you respect yourself? _____

_____

What are some of your greatest accomplishments? _____

_____

EMOTIONAL WELL-BEING

FEEL GOOD ABOUT YOURSELF

Step 4: Set Goals

Self-esteem is a critical component of your emotional well-being. Emotionally well people feel good about themselves. They are proud of who they are and what they have accomplished. Use the action planning tool below to deepen your sense of self-esteem. For your action plan, identify the self-esteem issues you want to change, set specific goals to achieve this change, and notice how much better you feel about yourself.

The behavior I want to change is _____

Goals need to be SMART:
Specific, **M**easureable, **A**ttainable, **R**ealistic and **T**ime-Specific

Goals	How I Will Measure This Goal	How Is This Goal Attainable and Realistic?	Time Deadline	How This Will Help Me
I need to stop worrying about what other people might think about me.	I will make note of each time I am able to ignore my own thoughts about what someone thinks.	Concentrate on positive things people say to me	One month from now	I will have less doubts about myself.

If you are having trouble identifying goals, consult TIPS, page 90.

EMOTIONAL WELL-BEING

FEEL GOOD ABOUT YOURSELF

Step 5: Monitor My Behavior – Pride

Pride is the emotional reaction you have about yourself and your accomplishments. What about yourself are you most proud of, and how can you develop deeper pride in yourself? One way is to begin to set goals for developing the pride within you so that it shows for everyone to see. In the chart below, set some goals to express your pride and watch your feelings for yourself grow. Periodic re-evaluation of your goals will help you feel better more quickly. Once you reach a goal, set new ones to improve or maintain what you already feel. Use a separate page for each change.

EXAMPLE:

My healthy behavior change   Be proud of my skills and talents

My goal   Teach music again because I love teaching people to play the piano

Date	My Accomplishment	How It Felt
1/1/2014	I advertised to teach music out of my home.	It felt great to again be teaching – my first love.

✂ -

Pride

My healthy behavior change _____

My goal _____

Date	My Accomplishment	How It Felt

(Continued on the next page)

EMOTIONAL WELL-BEING

FEEL GOOD ABOUT YOURSELF

Step 5: Monitor My Behavior – Image

Your image is the emotions generated from your internalized judgment of yourself. Unfortunately, this judgment is often based on false information or the perception of other people. Set some goals to enhance these emotions. The following guide is designed to do just that. By setting goals and working toward them, you will develop a better image of yourself. Keep reviewing these goals and setting new ones to work toward. Use a separate page for each change. Notice how much better you feel about yourself!

EXAMPLE:

My healthy behavior change *Stop worrying so much about what I look like*

My goal *Stop looking in the mirror at every opportunity I can*

Date	My Accomplishment	How It Felt
1/1/2014	I got dressed and glanced at the mirror once.	It felt good to walk by a store window and not check my reflection.

Image

My healthy behavior change _____

My goal _____

Date	My Accomplishment	How It Felt

(Continued on the next page)

EMOTIONAL WELL-BEING

FEEL GOOD ABOUT YOURSELF

Step 5: Monitor My Behavior – Outlook

Your outlook is directly related to how you feel about the positive emotions you feel as you go through your daily activities. People who feel good about themselves usually have a positive outlook, and vice versa! Now is the time to brighten your life's outlook. To get started, identify some goals that you can work toward. Monitor your progress and keep track of your results using the log below. Occasionally re-evaluate your results and develop new goals to improve your outlook even more. Use a separate page for each change.

EXAMPLE:

My healthy behavior change   Say "YES" to a healthy challenge

My goal   To take healthy risks

Date	My Accomplishment	How It Felt
1/1/2014	I volunteered to do something difficult at work.	It felt amazing when I accomplished it!

Outlook

My healthy behavior change _____

My goal _____

Date	My Accomplishment	How It Felt

(Continued on the next page)

EMOTIONAL WELL-BEING

FEEL GOOD ABOUT YOURSELF

Step 5: Monitor My Behavior – Self-Approval

As long as you like yourself, that's all that is important in developing and maintaining emotional well-being. Worrying about what others say about you or having your self-worth tied to others' opinions will keep you in emotional turmoil. To avoid having this happen to you, set some goals so that you worry less about the opinions of others. After setting goals, work hard to achieve them everyday. Use the chart below to watch your progress over time. Once you reach a goal, set new ones so that you feel even better about yourself. Use a separate page for each change.

EXAMPLE:

My healthy behavior change *Stop comparing myself to my neighbor Jane*

My goal *To stop shopping for the same things she purchases*

Date	My Accomplishment	How It Felt
1/1/2014	I went to the store to buy what I wanted.	I felt a sense of relief about not having to keep up with Jane.

✂--

Self-Approval

My healthy behavior change _____

My goal _____

Date	My Accomplishment	How It Felt

(Continued on the next page)

EMOTIONAL WELL-BEING

FEEL GOOD ABOUT YOURSELF

Step 5: Monitor My Behavior – Summary

In the table below, for each of the emotional categories please list some changes you want to make and how you expect your life to be different because of the changes.

Emotional Aspects of Wellness	Changes I Want to Make	Expected Results of This Behavior
Pride		
Image		
Outlook		
Self-Approval		

What did you learn about your self-esteem from this activity?

_____

_____

_____

EMOTIONAL WELL-BEING

FEEL GOOD ABOUT YOURSELF

Step 6: Reward Myself

When you feel good about yourself, it is easier to attain emotional well-being. It is interesting that when you begin to feel good about yourself, you will want to hang onto that feeling. To do so, you will need to reward yourself when you behave in a way that makes you feel good about yourself. People who reward themselves are more likely to work to achieve the same emotions again! The challenge is to decide what reward would motivate you to reach your goals. Your reward needs to be something that will give you the incentive to achieve your goals. It needs to be within your budget and something you'll be excited about. If you are buying yourself something, be sure your reward is something you wouldn't ordinarily buy or do. Brainstorm possible rewards.

- Rewards that would be meaningful to me _____
- Small rewards I could give myself _____
- Large rewards I could give myself _____
- Things that would not cost money and would be fun _____
- Rewards that I can afford and that would be fun _____
- Rewards that I enjoy alone _____
- Rewards I enjoy with people who support me _____

You deserve a pat on the back for the hard work you are completing in this session. Rewards help you to pay attention to your triumphs, not your setbacks. Rewards will create good feelings and propel you to want to work harder to reach your goals. Whenever you have completed or achieved one of your goals, treat yourself to one of the items on your list. You can also reward yourself by giving yourself positive affirmations when you have achieved a goal. Below are some samples. Cut them out and post in visible spots at home and work! If these don't work for your goal, write your own on sticky notes!

I won't compare myself to _____ anymore.	I am great!	I feel a sense of pride about myself.
I am capable of achieving my goals.	I am growing every day!	I have a positive outlook.
I am special.	My mind is full of gratitude for my life.	*I accept myself unconditionally.*

Gloria Steinem said, *"Self-esteem isn't everything; it's just that there's nothing without it."* What does this quote mean to you? _____

EMOTIONAL WELL-BEING

FEEL GOOD ABOUT YOURSELF

Step 7: Tips for Motivated Behavior Modification

Pride

- Make a list of all of your accomplishments from the past. These can be from work, leisure activities, family, school, or community – anything at all that you are proud of.

- Have a purpose to your life. People with high self-esteem are able to routinely set, update and revise their goals as they work toward them.

- Think about your life. What have you done that no other human being on earth, dead or alive, could have done?

Image

- Acknowledge and accept your positive qualities, but make an effort to grow in some way every day. It might require you to step outside your comfort zone and experience change and growth.

- Expect the best out of yourself without needing constant perfection.

- Take every opportunity to learn from your mistakes. Use this information to do better the next time.

Outlook

- Find a way to put a positive spin on your unfortunate situations. Look for ways to reframe these into positive situations – what you have gained – or how you might have grown.

- Understand that minor setbacks and bad times are only temporary and will pass.

- Live on the lighter side of life. Take time to laugh at yourself. Have fun with your family and your friends. You don't always have to take life so seriously.

Self-Approval

- Take positive risks and ignore your critics.

- Stop comparing yourself to others. This can be one of the most detrimental and fundamental roadblocks to high self-esteem.

- Learn to get past the opinions of others. These opinions can influence your beliefs, behaviors, emotions and self-esteem.

- Stay solid in what you know about yourself and your self-expectations.

SECTION VI
ACCEPT CHANGE

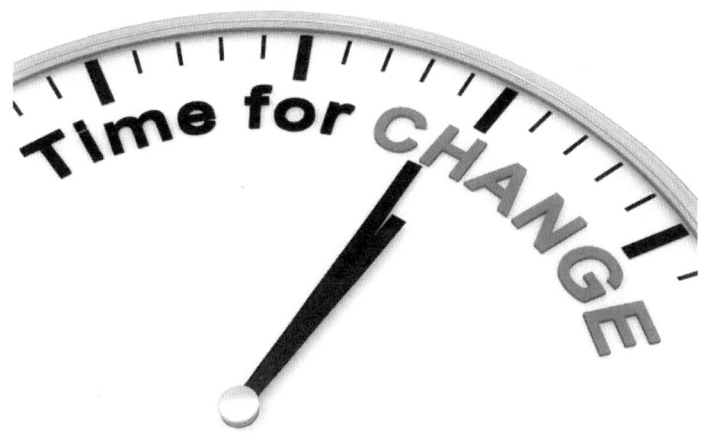

*"If you don't like something change it;
if you can't change it,
change the way you think about it."*

~ Mary Engelbreit

Name _____

Date _____

EMOTIONAL WELL-BEING

EMOTIONAL WELL-BEING

ACCEPT CHANGE

Step 1: Self-Assessment Introduction and Directions

Emotionally-well people go with the flow in times of change. One of the best ways to deal with change in your life is to learn how to effectively cope with it. People have varying levels of skills for coping with change, as well as preferred methods for coping with it.

This self-assessment is designed to help you understand how effective you are in preventing and coping with change. It will assess your skills for coping with change. Read each statement carefully. Circle the number of the response under the column True, Somewhat True or Not True that shows how descriptive each statement is of you. Do NOT pay attention to the number itself, just the column. Please answer all the questions to the best of your ability using the following scale:

True   **Somewhat True**   **Not True**

In the following example, the circled 2 indicates that the statement is **Somewhat True** for the person completing the scale.

	True	Somewhat True	Not True

When I'm in a time of change ...

I engage in wishful thinking	1	(2)	3

This is not a test and there are no right or wrong answers. Do not spend too much time thinking about your answers. Your initial response will be the most true for you. Be sure to respond to every statement.

Turn the page and complete the Self-Assessment

EMOTIONAL WELL-BEING

ACCEPT CHANGE

Step 1: Self-Assessment

	True	Somewhat True	Not True
When I'm in a time of change ...			
I engage in wishful thinking	1	2	3
I find it difficult to stop and/or correct my self-talk.	1	2	3
I sometimes question my worth as a human being.	1	2	3
I can alter my expectations to match the changes occurring	3	2	1
I have many pessimistic thoughts	1	2	3
I know how to monitor my negative self-talk	3	2	1
I often say things like "I can't do this"	1	2	3
I can see the opportunities in a new situation	3	2	1

I. TOTAL = _____

When I'm in a time of change ...			
I often have a hard time coping	1	2	3
I manage the stress associated with it well	3	2	1
I get angry	1	2	3
I have religious and/or spiritual beliefs that comfort me.	3	2	1
I use relaxation techniques to relax my body	3	2	1
I have an adequate support system to help manage my stress.	3	2	1
I fail to take care of myself and my personal needs	1	2	3
I am assertive in asking for what I want	3	2	1

II. TOTAL = _____

When I'm in a time of change ...			
I often try to control the things I cannot control	1	2	3
I focus on the things in my life I can do something about.	3	2	1
I set new goals for myself and work toward them	3	2	1
If one path does not work, I try another	3	2	1
I see the world as perfect as it is	3	2	1
I let go of things beyond my control	3	2	1
I am overly sensitive of critical statements from others	1	2	3
I "go with the flow"	3	2	1

III. TOTAL = _____

Go to the Scoring Directions on the next page

EMOTIONAL WELL-BEING

ACCEPT CHANGE

Step 1: Self-Assessment Scoring Directions

Add the numbers you circled for each section on the scale and write that score on the line marked TOTAL at the end of the section. Then transfer those totals to the spaces below:

I. Realistic TOTAL = _____
Your ability to alter your negative thinking, see change more realistically, and be more optimistic during times of change.

II. Wellness TOTAL = _____
Your ability to take care of yourself and relax and manage stress during times of change.

III. Control TOTAL = _____
Your ability to take positive action, go with the flow of life and try to control only those things that you are able to control during times of change.

Next, add your three totals to get your Grand Total = _____

Profile Interpretation

Individual Scales Scores	Grand Total	Result	Indications
Scores from 19 to 24	57 to 72	High	If you score in the high range, you tend to be effective in accepting change and going with the flow.
Scores from 14 to 18	40 to 56	Moderate	If you score in the moderate range, you tend to be somewhat effective in accepting change and going with the flow.
Scores from 8 to 13	24 to 39	Low	If you score in the low range, you are not very effective in accepting change and going with the flow.

EMOTIONAL WELL-BEING

ACCEPT CHANGE

Step 2: Recognize and Develop a Support System

Some people are better than others at accepting change and going with the flow of life. You will want to have these people as part of your support system to help you in your efforts to accept change. Identify those people in your life who are good at accepting change and ask them if they would be willing to support you in your efforts to grow in this area. Complete the following table with people who might be able to support you with accepting change as a part of life and helping you to "go with the flow" more often.

Supporter	How This Person Can Support Me	How I Can Contact This Person
My therapist	By giving me someone I trust to talk to when I need help	Phone: 000-000-0000

Keep this list handy. Call, email or text when you need support.

ACCEPT CHANGE

Step 3: Keep a Journal

Change is an event that everyone must endure. A famous quote, "change is the only constant," suggests that you are going to encounter more changes in your life. Now is the time to explore what you feel about change and how it affects your emotions. The following journaling questions will help you to explore how change affects your emotional well-being.

What is the biggest change coming up in your personal life?

_____
_____
_____

How did you react to this change?

_____
_____
_____

What is the biggest change happening in your professional life?

_____
_____
_____

How did you react to this change?

_____
_____
_____

Why does change frustrate you?

_____
_____
_____

How can you begin to see the opportunities in the changes in life?

_____
_____
_____

EMOTIONAL WELL-BEING

ACCEPT CHANGE

Step 4: Set Goals

People in the midst of change often feel frustrated, angry, anxious, and envious. Think about how change makes you feel as you develop some goals that will help you "go with the flow" more effectively. Well-conceived action plans can help you to stay motivated as you work toward your goals. For your action plan, identify both the behavior you want to change and specific goals, or smaller goals required to reach your ultimate goals for accepting change and dealing with it effectively.

The behavior I want to change is _____

Goals need to be SMART:
Specific, **M**easureable, **A**ttainable, **R**ealistic and **T**ime-Specific

Goals	How I Will Measure This Goal	How is This Goal Attainable and Realistic?	Time Deadline	How This Will Help Me
To realize I can't control every situation	How often I get angry when situations change	Yes, if I work on it and control everyone and everything.	My birthday	I will experience less stress and anger and others will not be upset with me.

If you are having trouble identifying goals, consult TIPS, page 106.

EMOTIONAL WELL-BEING

ACCEPT CHANGE

Step 5: Monitor My Behavior – Realistic

Pride is the emotional reaction you have about yourself and your accomplishments. What about yourself are you most proud of, and how can you develop deeper pride in yourself? One way is to begin to set goals for developing the pride within you so that it shows for everyone to see. In the chart that follows, set some goals to express your pride and watch your feelings for yourself grow. Periodic re-evaluation of your goals will help you feel better more quickly. Once you reach a goal, set new ones to improve or maintain what you already feel. Use a separate page for each change.

EXAMPLE:

My healthy behavior change   *I want to limit my negative self-talk.*

My goal   *Stop the internal chatter in my mind*

Date	My Accomplishment	How It Felt
1/1/2014	I listened to a guided imagery tape.	I felt much calmer throughout the day.

✂ -

Realistic

My healthy behavior change _____

My goal _____

Date	My Accomplishment	How It Felt

(Continued on the next page)

EMOTIONAL WELL-BEING

ACCEPT CHANGE

Step 5: Monitor My Behavior – Realistic (Continued)

Answer the following questions to learn more about what you think and how you feel in times of change.

In times of change what negative thoughts go through your mind?

_____

_____

_____

Identify an opportunity you can see hidden in a recent change.

_____

_____

_____

How can you get a more realistic perspective about your life?

_____

_____

_____

How can you be less judgmental in new situations?

_____

_____

_____

What is the silver lining of a change you are going through?

_____

_____

_____

EMOTIONAL WELL-BEING

ACCEPT CHANGE

Step 5: Monitor My Behavior – Wellness

It is important to take care of yourself while you are going through changes. Your ability to cope with stress during change often determines how effective you are in managing the change. Personal wellness is fairly easy to track. Through the chart below, you will monitor your progress toward being able to emotionally deal with change. You should re-evaluate your goals as you develop more confidence in this process. Once you reach your goal(s), set new ones to improve or maintain what you have already achieved. Use a separate page for each change.

EXAMPLE:

My healthy behavior change   I'm taking more time for myself.

My goal   To be calmer and more patient

Date	My Accomplishment	How It Felt
1/1/2014	I had a massage.	I felt relaxed and it felt wonderful.

Wellness

My healthy behavior change _____

My goal _____

Date	My Accomplishment	How It Felt

(Continued on the next page)

EMOTIONAL WELL-BEING

ACCEPT CHANGE

Step 5: Monitor My Behavior – Wellness *(Continued)*

Answer the following questions to gauge your effectiveness in handling the stress of change.

What was your last stressful change?
_____
_____
_____

How did you handle it?
_____
_____
_____

During the change, how did it affect you?
_____
_____
_____

What could you have done differently?
_____
_____
_____

Once the change was in place, how did it affect you?
_____
_____
_____

How do your religious and/or spiritual beliefs help you in times of change?
_____
_____
_____

ACCEPT CHANGE

Step 5: Monitor My Behavior – Control

Emotionally well people make positive choices in regard to what they can control, and do not worry about things they cannot control. They also do not try to control the changes they encounter. They are able to simply go with the flow of change and make the best of it. Monitoring your progress toward your goals of not trying to control everything, and everyone, will help to reinforce your behavior. Periodic re-evaluations promote your success. Once you reach your goal(s), set new ones to improve or maintain what you have already achieved. Use a separate page for each change.

EXAMPLE:

My healthy behavior change   I'm going to try not to fix everybody else's issues.

My goal   Let people take care of their own lives

Date	My Accomplishment	How It Felt
1/1/2014	I did not give directions when a friend was driving.	I felt relaxed knowing that we'd get there, even if it wasn't the fastest way.

Control

My healthy behavior change _____

My goal _____

Date	My Accomplishment	How It Felt

(Continued on the next page)

EMOTIONAL WELL-BEING

ACCEPT CHANGE

Step 5: Monitor My Behavior – Control *(Continued)*

Answer the following questions about your attempts to control the changes inherent in life.

In what ways do you expect the world to be perfect?
___
___
___

How does this affect you?
___
___
___

Who and what do you try to control?
___
___
___

How does that person feel about it?
___
___
___

How can you change this?
___
___
___

What types of things CAN you control in life?
___
___
___

EMOTIONAL WELL-BEING

ACCEPT CHANGE

Step 6: Reward Myself

Emotionally well people are able to overcome the various negative feelings that are associated with change, view change positively, and be flexible and spontaneous in their reaction to change. When you are able to accomplish this, remember to reward yourself! This will motivate you to duplicate this behavior more. The challenge is to decide what reward would motivate you to reach your goal. Your reward needs to be something that will give you the incentive to achieve your goals. It needs to be within your budget and something you'll be excited about. If you are buying yourself something, be sure your reward is something you wouldn't ordinarily buy or do. Brainstorm possible rewards.

- Rewards that would be meaningful to me _____
- Small rewards I could give myself _____
- Large rewards I could give myself _____
- Things that would not cost money and would be fun _____
- Rewards that I can afford and that would be fun _____
- Rewards that I enjoy alone _____
- Rewards I enjoy with people who support me _____

You deserve a pat on the back for the hard work you are completing in this session. Rewards help you to pay attention to your triumphs, not your setbacks. Rewards will create good feelings and propel you to want to work harder to reach your goals. Whenever you have completed or achieved one of your goals, treat yourself to one of the items on your list. You can also reward yourself by giving yourself positive affirmations when you have achieved a goal. Below are some samples. Cut them out and post in visible spots at home and work! If these don't work for your goal, write your own on sticky notes!

I can live with uncertainty!	I cannot control everything.	Things in life change and I can adapt!
I can manage the stress of change.	I am proud of myself for trying!	I am willing to try new things.
Change can energize me!	I see opportunities everywhere!	*I am able to stretch my comfort zone.*

"Life is a series of natural and spontaneous changes. Don't resist them – that only creates sorrow. Let reality be reality. Let things flow naturally forward in whatever way they like."

~Lao-Tzu

EMOTIONAL WELL-BEING

ACCEPT CHANGE

Step 7: Tips for Motivated Behavior Modification

Realistic

- Remember that life changes bring with them a variety of purposes and opportunities. For your own knowledge, review how purpose and opportunities have changed your life.

- As new situations arise, try not to be judgmental. Look at each situation as realistically and as openly as you can.

- Monitor the thoughts that keep going through your head. Although your initial thoughts about change may be negative, you can change them to be more positive.

- Open up to potential opportunities. Be willing to do whatever is necessary to turn opportunities into realities.

- Remember that things you feel are very important now will not seem as important as time goes by.

Wellness

- Take care of yourself by eating healthy foods, getting enough sleep, exercising, and eliminating or start minimizing your use of alcohol and tobacco products.

- Use techniques for managing the stress of change by meditating, using progressive relaxation techniques, and staying in the present.

- Nurture yourself as much as possible. You may want to treat yourself to a massage, enjoy a walk in the woods, take time to read a good book, or pack and eat a picnic lunch in a park.

Control

- Stop being so afraid to make mistakes. All people make mistakes, but you need to reflect on your behaviors and learn from them so you do not repeat the same behaviors.

- Let go of trying to control the outcomes of your actions and trust your intuition.

- Be willing to live with a certain amount of uncertainty. By wanting to know how everything is going to turn out, you will begin to worry unnecessarily. Learn to trust the process.

- Review the Serenity Prayer.

    Grant me the serenity to accept the things I cannot change,

    The courage to change the things I can,

    and wisdom to know the difference.

SECTION VII
ENJOY LIFE, LAUGH and HAVE FUN

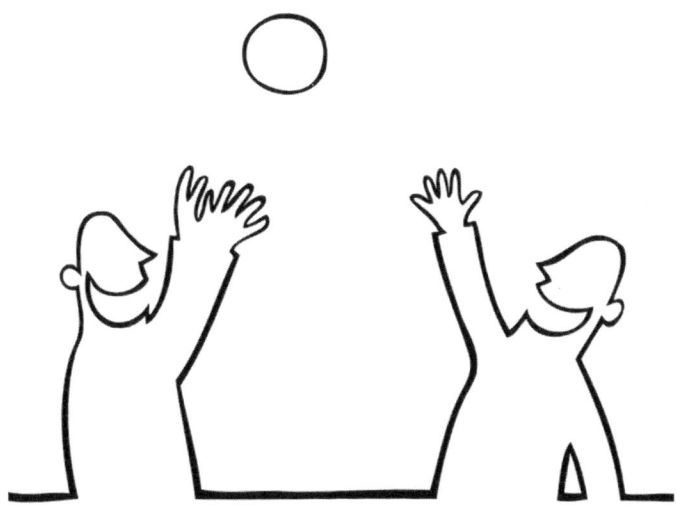

"Life is too important to be taken seriously."

~ Oscar Wilde

Name _____

Date _____

EMOTIONAL WELL-BEING

ENJOY LIFE, LAUGH and HAVE FUN

Step 1: Self-Assessment Introduction and Directions

Research has shown that the health benefits of laughter are enormous. Laughter can reduce stress and relieve pain. One study showed that healthy children may laugh 400 times a day but adults tend to laugh only 16 times a day. By maintaining a sense of humor, stressors feel less stressful. Tension will melt with a good laugh.

This self-assessment will help you identify how much of your life is filled with joy, laughter and fun activities. Circle the YES-NO answer that describes you.

In the following example, the circled NO indicates that the statement is not descriptive of the person completing the inventory.

I stop and "smell the roses" . . . . YES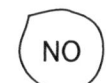

This is not a test. Since there are no right or wrong answers, do not spend too much time thinking about your answers. Be sure to respond to every statement.

Turn the page and complete the Self-Assessment

EMOTIONAL WELL-BEING

ENJOY LIFE, LAUGH and HAVE FUN

Step 1: Self-Assessment

I stop and "smell the roses"	YES	NO
I savor life's joys	YES	NO
I relish ordinary experiences	YES	NO
I am open to the beauty around me	YES	NO
I replay happy life events in my mind	YES	NO
I share successes and accomplishments with others	YES	NO
I often reminisce happy times with family and friends	YES	NO
I love music – singing, dancing, playing, listening	YES	NO
I take discovery walks	YES	NO
I take time to slow down and enjoy life	YES	NO
I spend time with fun, playful people	YES	NO
I feel pleasure by seeing children play, or playing with them	YES	NO
I like to play card and board games with others	YES	NO
I watch funny sitcoms	YES	NO
I try to pick out funny movies to view	YES	NO
I keep a gratitude journal	YES	NO
I enjoy whatever I am doing at the moment	YES	NO
I have enjoyable things to do in my leisure time	YES	NO
I spend my time with interesting people	YES	NO
I laugh at situations rather than complain	YES	NO

TOTAL 1 = _____

(Self-assessment continued on the next page)

EMOTIONAL WELL-BEING

ENJOY LIFE, LAUGH and HAVE FUN

Step 1: Self-Assessment *(continued)*

I have friends and family who make me laugh.	YES	NO
I laugh aloud when reading humorous books.	YES	NO
I laugh aloud at funny movies, in the theater or at home.	YES	NO
Laughter relaxes by body	YES	NO
I can laugh at ridiculous situations	YES	NO
I feel closer to people when we share a good belly laugh.	YES	NO
When I laugh I feel less stressed	YES	NO
If I laugh at something I can't get angry.	YES	NO
I agree, laughter is the best medicine	YES	NO
Laughter dissolves my anxieties	YES	NO
I love to laugh with other people.	YES	NO
I like the sound of laughter	YES	NO
Sometimes I laugh so hard, tears come to my eyes.	YES	NO
I have friends and family who make me laugh.	YES	NO
I enjoy hearing or reading a good joke.	YES	NO
I have certain family members that I like to be with because of their sense of humor	YES	NO
I have a great sense of humor.	YES	NO
When I feel like having fun I go out with friends who have a sense of humor	YES	NO
I love to laugh, but never at anyone's expense	YES	NO
I like jokes, but not the kind that make fun of anyone or any culture.	YES	NO

TOTAL 2 = _____

(Self-assessment continued on the next page)

EMOTIONAL WELL-BEING

ENJOY LIFE, LAUGH and HAVE FUN

Step 1: Self-Assessment *(continued)*

I like to be silly sometimes	YES	NO
I often see the ridiculous side of situations	YES	NO
I enjoy new situations	YES	NO
I engage in leisure activities just to relax	YES	NO
I am able to lighten up when necessary	YES	NO
I am able to easily have fun regardless of the situation	YES	NO
I find ways to have an enjoyable time, even when I'm miserable	YES	NO
I don't need substances or drugs to have a good time	YES	NO
I like to get out of my comfort zone, if it's safe	YES	NO
I like to play or watch a sport	YES	NO
I love to play with a pet, mine or anyone else's	YES	NO
I like to socialize with fun friends	YES	NO
I like to look at old photos that remind me of great times	YES	NO
I make sure that I schedule in fun time into my week	YES	NO
I like to explore my artistic side	YES	NO
I enjoy looking "outside of the box"	YES	NO
I like an adventure	YES	NO
I am a healthy risk taker	YES	NO
I don't mind losing as long as the game is fun	YES	NO
I like to be spontaneous	YES	NO

TOTAL 3 = _____

Go to the Scoring Directions on the next page

EMOTIONAL WELL-BEING

ENJOY LIFE, LAUGH and HAVE FUN

Step 1: Self-Assessment Scoring Directions

The Enjoy Life, Laugh & Have Fun Self-Assessment is designed to measure how much pleasure you have in your day-to-day life. For each of the sections on the self-assessment you completed, count the YES responses you circled for each of the three sections. Place that total on the line marked TOTAL at the end of each section.

Then, transfer your totals to the spaces below:

TOTAL 1 = _____ Enjoy Life

TOTAL 2 = _____ Laugh

TOTAL 3 = _____ Have Fun

Add these three scores (you will get a number from 0 to 60) to get your grand total and place that number below:

GRAND TOTAL = _____

Profile Interpretation

Individual Scales Scores	Total Scales Scores	Result	Indications
Scores from 14 to 20	Scores from 41 to 60	High	You have definitely developed the ability to enjoy life, have fun and laugh.
Scores from 7 to 13	Scores from 20 to 40	Moderate	You have somewhat developed the ability to enjoy life, have fun and laugh.
Scores from 0 to 6	Scores from 0 to 19	Low	You have not yet developed the ability to enjoy life, have fun and laugh.

Go to the Scale Descriptions on the next page

EMOTIONAL WELL-BEING

ENJOY LIFE, LAUGH and HAVE FUN

Step 1: Self-Assessment Descriptions

Enjoy Life – People scoring high on this self-assessment tend to take every opportunity to enjoy life. They live in the present but also take time to reminisce about good times from the past. They enjoy ordinary life experiences and take time to enjoy the beauties of their environment. They are able to keep things in perspective, manage their stress, and hang out with other people who enjoy life. They think in a positive way, count their blessings, find humor in their life and are willing to step out of their comfort zone.

Laugh – People scoring high on this self-assessment tend to enjoy laughing in life. They smile a lot and enjoy laughing through reading humorous books, seeing silly movies, and telling jokes. They have a good sense of humor and are able to laugh at themselves without getting defensive. They are aware that laughter connects them with others (it is more contagious than a cough, sneeze or sniffle), and know that it is a great form of stress relief and relief from pain.

Have Fun – People scoring high on this self-assessment tend to be able to enjoy having fun. They enjoy new and novel situations and are able to find ways to have fun at work and at home. They enjoy leisure activities and are able to lighten up when times get stressful. They play and socialize with fun, optimistic friends and enjoy hobbies and passions.

The following activities are designed to help you begin enjoying life, having fun and laughing. Please complete all of the following exercises.

Step 2: Recognize and Develop a Support System

If you are like most people, you have many people in your life you seem to really enjoy life, laugh a lot, and not take everything so seriously. Think about who those people are and how they could help you to develop the positive emotions that accompany enjoyment and contentment in life. In order to be able to make the behavioral changes you desire, you need to recognize your current support system and identify who might be helpful to you. Not every supportive person in your life will fit this bill, so now is the time to identify those who can support you in your efforts to grow. Complete the following table with people who might support you in living a more joyful life.

Supporter	How This Person Can Support Me	How I Can Contact This Person
My friend who has a more fun-loving personality than me.	*She can keep reminding me that there's more to life than work.*	*phone or text 135-7913 email Friend@xyz.com*

Keep this list handy. Call, email or text when you need support.

EMOTIONAL WELL-BEING

ENJOY LIFE, LAUGH and HAVE FUN

Step 3: Keep a Journal

You too can begin to enjoy life more! You may be asking how this is possible. The first step is to explore what brings you enjoyment and makes you laugh. The following journaling questions are designed to help you think carefully about the joy in your life. Answer them honestly and you will have insight into what makes you feel more satisfied and content in life.

What or who brings you the most joy in your life? Explain.

_____
_____
_____

What is your idea of fun?

_____
_____
_____

What types of activities are fun for you?

_____
_____
_____

When or with whom do you find yourself laughing the most? Explain.

_____
_____
_____

How can you find more time to spend with those people?

_____
_____
_____

Identify some new activities that might bring you joy in the future.

_____
_____
_____

EMOTIONAL WELL-BEING

ENJOY LIFE, LAUGH and HAVE FUN

Step 4: Set Goals

The next step in enjoying life more is to set specific goals that will bring more enjoyment and laughter into your life. The action plan that follows will help you to achieve your goals by keeping you motivated. For your action plan, identify both the behaviors that will bring you enjoyment, and then set specific goals, or smaller goals that can help keep you motivated until you reach your goals of living a life with more joy, fun & laughter in it.

The behavior I want to change is _____

Goals need to be SMART:
Specific, **M**easureable, **A**ttainable, **R**ealistic and **T**ime-Specific

Goals	How I Will Measure This Goal	How Is This Goal Attainable and Realistic?	Time Deadline	How This Will Help Me
I will stop and enjoy my accomplishments before hurrying to get to the next task.	The number of times I reward myself for a job well done.	Yes, if I just slow down and enjoy life.	Immediately	I will be more appreciative of my life.

If you are having trouble identifying goals, consult TIPS, page 124.

EMOTIONAL WELL-BEING

ENJOY LIFE, LAUGH and HAVE FUN

Step 5: Monitor My Behavior – Enjoy Life

"How can I enjoy life more?" is a question that people have asked for centuries. Now you can live a more enjoyable life by identifying goals to help you enjoy life more. In the log that follows, identify some of the goals you have that will bring you more joy and laughter. This can be anything from getting a new job to watching more comedies you like on television. Monitor your progress toward your goals by keeping track of your behaviors below. Periodic re-evaluations support your success. Once you reach your goal(s), set new ones to improve or maintain what you have already achieved. Use a separate page for each change.

EXAMPLE:

My healthy behavior change   Spend time with my children's activities

My goal   To enjoy my children more

Date	My Accomplishment	How It Felt
1/1/2014	I went to my son's soccer game.	I enjoyed myself and was so proud of him.

Enjoy Life

My healthy behavior change _____

My goal _____

Date	My Accomplishment	How It Felt

(Continued on the next page)

EMOTIONAL WELL-BEING

ENJOY LIFE, LAUGH and HAVE FUN

Step 5: Monitor My Behavior – Enjoy Life (Continued)

In the Table that follows, write about some of the things you can do to begin living your life more, how it will change your mindset and help you emotionally.

Ways I Will Try to Enjoy My Life	How I Will Need to Change My Mindset	How This Will Help Me Emotionally

How will enjoying life make you a more content person?_____
_____
_____

EMOTIONAL WELL-BEING

ENJOY LIFE, LAUGH and HAVE FUN

Step 5: Monitor My Behavior – Laugh

Laughter has been shown to positively affect people who are sick or depressed, and can definitely enhance your emotional well-being. You can take advantage of this tool for developing a more light-hearted approach to life. Laughter is something that you can fairly easily track during your week. In the chart that follows, monitor your progress in laughing more. Keeping track of these laughs through logs will help you determine where you are at given times. Periodic re-evaluations are vital for your success in your developing a more humorous attitude. Once you reach your goal(s), set new ones to improve or maintain what you have already achieved. Use a separate page for each change.

EXAMPLE:

My healthy behavior change To laugh more

My goal To take time each day to read a joke and laugh

Date	My Accomplishment	How It Felt
1/1/2014	I bought a joke-a-day calendar.	It felt good to laugh and felt even better when co-workers stopped by to hear the joke-of-the-day.

- -

Laugh

My healthy behavior change _____

My goal _____

Date	My Accomplishment	How It Felt

(Continued on the next page)

EMOTIONAL WELL-BEING

ENJOY LIFE, LAUGH and HAVE FUN

Step 5: Monitor My Behavior – Laugh *(Continued)*

Complete the following questions to better assess your humor quotient.

What makes you laugh? Explain.
_____
_____
_____

Who makes you laugh? _____
How? _____
_____
_____

Who do you make laugh? _____
How? _____
_____
_____

What is the value of laughter in your life?
_____
_____
_____

How do you, or can you, use laughter to lighten up some tough situations?
_____
_____
_____

Guess how many times a day you think you laugh? _____
Tomorrow, count the times you actually laugh and see how close you came to guessing correctly. When you're counting, no fair counting fake laughs!

What television show or movie do you watch to get a good laugh?
_____
_____
_____

Compare your responses with others. You all might get some good ideas.

ENJOY LIFE, LAUGH and HAVE FUN

Step 5: Monitor My Behavior – Have Fun

To have fun sounds easy, doesn't it? It does, but some people, for whatever reasons, are unable to have fun in life. To begin having more fun in your life, set some "have fun" goals. Fun seems like something that you do not have to set goals for, but rather something you just go and do. For some people that is the case. For others, it helps to set goals to work toward. Use the chart that follows to set "have fun" goals and monitoring your progress toward these goals. Keeping track of your behaviors through logs will help you determine your progress at given times. Once you reach your goal(s), set new ones to improve or maintain what you have already achieved. Use a separate page for each change.

EXAMPLE:

My healthy behavior change   To be more fun to be around rather than always griping

My goal   To have less stress in the workplace

Date	My Accomplishment	How It Felt
1/1/2014	I brought some crossword puzzles that we do together at break-time.	I felt accomplished because it helped me and my co-workers to have more positive interactions.

- -

Have Fun

My healthy behavior change _____

My goal _____

Date	My Accomplishment	How It Felt

(Continued on the next page)

EMOTIONAL WELL-BEING

ENJOY LIFE, LAUGH and HAVE FUN

Step 5: Monitor My Behavior – Have Fun (Continued)

What present activities do you find fun and want to do more of?

_____
_____
_____

What activities do you not find fun and would like to do away with?

_____
_____
_____

What new activities sound like fun to you, that you would like to try?

_____
_____
_____

Have you ever seen the ridiculous part of a stressful situation? Describe the situation.

_____
_____
_____

Were you able to laugh about that situation at the time or afterwards. Explain.

_____
_____
_____

EMOTIONAL WELL-BEING

ENJOY LIFE, LAUGH and HAVE FUN

Step 6: Reward Myself

Rewarding yourself for having fun seems redundant. In actuality, providing yourself with rewards for having healthy fun will help to reinforce the behavior and ensure you engage in the behavior again. The challenge is to decide what reward would motivate you to reach your life enjoyment goals. Your reward needs to be something that will give you the incentive to achieve your goals. It needs to be within your budget and something you'll be excited about. If you are buying yourself something, be sure your reward is something you wouldn't ordinarily buy or do. Brainstorm possible rewards.

- Rewards that would be meaningful to me _____
- Small rewards I could give myself _____
- Large rewards I could give myself _____
- Things that would not cost money and would be fun _____
- Rewards that I can afford and that would be fun _____
- Rewards that I enjoy alone _____
- Rewards I enjoy with people who support me _____

You deserve a pat on the back for the hard work you are completing in this session. Rewards help you to pay attention to your triumphs, not your setbacks. Rewards will create good feelings and propel you to want to work harder to reach your goals. Whenever you have completed or achieved one of your goals, treat yourself to one of the items on your list. You can also reward yourself by giving yourself positive affirmations when you have achieved a goal. Below are some samples. Cut them out and post in visible spots at home and work! If these don't work for your goal, write your own on sticky notes!

I want to have more fun!	I can laugh at myself.	I can make light of difficult situations.
I like being with people who have a good sense of humor.	*I can find funniness in stressful situations.*	*I enjoy my life.*
Play is important for adults too!	A good belly laugh is a good thing!	*I will stop and smell the roses.*

"Your sense of humor is one of the most powerful tools you have to make certain that your daily mood and emotional state support good health."

~ Paul E. McGhee, Ph.D

EMOTIONAL WELL-BEING

ENJOY LIFE, LAUGH and HAVE FUN

Step 7: Tips for Motivated Behavior Modification

Enjoy Life

- Get out of the ruts that are inhabiting your life.
- Experience the enjoyment of going to new places, doing different things and meeting new people.
- Take healthy risks.
- Make time to socialize with family and friends.
- Be spontaneous and flexible in your approach to life.
- Enjoy now! Do not anticipate happiness sometime in the future.
- Have an adventure-a-day (even if it's going to the store with someone).
- If possible, let go of friends and activities that you do not enjoy.

Laugh

- Surround yourself with people who are funny.
- Don't be so serious all the time.
- Take time to be silly.
- Look for the ridiculous side of situations.
- Take the time to enjoy humorous movies, plays, books, videos and people.
- Think back to humorous past situations in your life and enjoy a good laugh.

Have Fun

- Continue to engage in playful activities. Play is important for children and adults.
- Forget about the results and focus on the journey. For example, if you decide to write a book, you don't need to publish it, just write for the love of writing.
- Engage in creative activities such as scrapbooking, writing, singing, dancing, etc.
- Find ways to have more fun in your life.
- Eliminate those things in your life that are not fun or that others think are fun, but you don't.

Whole Person Associates is the leading publisher of training resources for professionals who empower people to create and maintain healthy lifestyles. Our creative resources will help you work effectively with your clients in the areas of stress management, wellness promotion, mental health and life skills.

Please visit us at our web site: **www.wholeperson.com**. You can check out our entire line of products, place an order, request our print catalog, and sign up for our monthly special notifications.

Whole Person Associates

800-247-6789